# Getting Rid of Cybersickness

Andras Kemeny · Jean-Rémy Chardonnet ·
Florent Colombet

# Getting Rid of Cybersickness

In Virtual Reality, Augmented Reality,
and Simulators

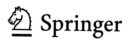
Springer

Andras Kemeny
Institut Image
Arts et Métiers Institute of Technology
Chalon-sur-Saône, France

Technocenter
Renault Group
Guyancourt, France

Florent Colombet
Technocenter
Renault Group
Guyancourt, France

Jean-Rémy Chardonnet
Institut Image
Arts et Métiers Institute of Technology
Chalon-sur-Saône, France

ISBN 978-3-030-59341-4      ISBN 978-3-030-59342-1   (eBook)
https://doi.org/10.1007/978-3-030-59342-1

This Springer imprint is published by the registered company Springer Nature Switzerland AG
The registered company address is: Gewerbestrasse 11, 6330 Cham, Switzerland

# Preface

The first Virtual Reality (VR) helmet was designed in 1968 by Ivan Sutherland, though at that time it was barely displaying wired frame images, as high-quality Computer-Generated Imagery (CGI) became available only from the mid-1980s. The first VR videogame was introduced in 1985 by Nintendo, through Virtual Boy, an innovative, though relatively simple VR system. Unfortunately, it was a major failure, largely due to motion sickness, experienced by the gamers. Kaiser Optical Systems then proposed VR helmets for professional use in 1998: ProView 30 for 8 K\$ and ProView 60 for 12 K\$. The latter was applied to driving simulators, exposing to not only drivability problems (i.e., transport delay between actions and maneuvering results), but also motion sickness, especially in round points, inducing sharp rotational accelerations, a critical issue in VR navigation.

More recently, Facebook acquired Oculus for US \$2 billion in early 2014 and delivered helmets to early developers and adopters, which again presented the same sickness effects that had previously limited the real development of public use of video games. Interestingly, Microsoft's HoloLens Augmented Reality (AR) helmet, available for developers in early 2016 and the Magic Leap (valued at US \$4.5 billion at the end of that year), another AR helmet available in the market in early 2019, do not seem to meet the same problems, thanks to the presence of real-world visual references, as discussed in Sects. 1.2 and 4.6. Increasingly, millions of helmets are delivered to public customers, especially Gear VR, codeveloped with Google and commercialized in a pack for Galaxy S7 users. The promised success for extensive public use is nevertheless not at rendezvous and motion or cybersickness or Virtual Reality Induced Sickness Effects (VRISE) is still a significant issue.

The first CAVE (Cave Automatic Virtual Environment—immersive 3D room) installations arrived in the early 1990s. Surprisingly, in immersive rooms, such as CAVEs—one can see his or her body, which is one of the advantages of Augmented Reality (AR) helmets, as it allows for reduced cybersickness. Unnatural navigation, such as walking, using joysticks, may also pose problems and recent studies have described comparable sickness effects. If the physical environment is sufficiently visible, AR helmets provide stable visual references and thus less critical situations. However, since our world is becoming more and more immersive, we can expect

VRISE to become a significant social issue if its adverse effects are not corrected in the next future through the integration of smart technologies.

Why is VR inducing these sickness effects? Would that be because of the difference from the real world? Several studies from the early 1990s have already demonstrated the impact of the field of view on scale perception, for example. The more realistic is the produced virtual environment, the more these effects may be disturbing if some of the perceptual cues are mismatching. This phenomenon is one of the main subjects of the present book, and previous theoretical explanations are discussed in detail in Chap. 2. From them, it can be inferred that one of the main reasons for this phenomenon are the discrepancies between the presented visual and vestibular cues. When moving virtually, such as navigating using a joystick, the image of the seen visual world also moves on the retina of the eyes following the movement, while the inner ears, responsible for the person's equilibrium communicate no movement. The temporal discrepancy between these cues is frequent, when images are displayed with some delays.

In addition to these multi-sensorial causes, discrepancies between the fundamental elementary visual depth cues, namely, binocular vision (mostly though not always provided by stereoscopy) and accommodation can cause highly disturbing effects when the induced distance information is significantly different.

There are many studies about these phenomena and some offer solutions to avoid them, a few are simplistic, such as teleportation (cinematic or precision blink), others technological, such as light field systems. These solutions form another subject of the present book. Nevertheless, VR navigation is still difficult to avoid without inducing some motion sickness effects if one wants to keep a free hand in motion and high-quality image generation.

Many business analyses predict the quick development of VR in our professional and personal lives. Several, though, flag the possible deception of users as an issue, and some even as a major obstacle in an extensive deployment of VR in everyday life. Hence, the present book intends to contribute to understanding how efficiently our brains produce a coherent and rich representation of the perceived outside world and to the challenging task of helping VR techniques to evolve toward equally efficient views of the world.

The book also outlines the social consequences, from engineering design to autonomous vehicle motion sickness, through video games, with the hope of providing an insight into VR sickness induced by the emerging immersive technologies.

Andras Kemeny
Institut Image, Arts et Métiers
Institute of Technology
Chalon-sur-Saône, France

Technocenter, Renault Group
Guyancourt, France

# Contents

**1 Introduction** ....................................................... 1
  1.1 Virtual Reality, Augmented Reality, Mixed Reality:
     Definitions ...................................................... 3
     1.1.1  Virtual Reality ........................................ 3
     1.1.2  Augmented Reality ................................... 3
     1.1.3  Mixed Reality ........................................ 4
     1.1.4  What About XR? ..................................... 4
  1.2 Cybersickness, VR Sickness, Simulator Sickness, Motion
     Sickness, and VRISE: Definitions ............................ 5
     1.2.1  Definition ............................................ 5
     1.2.2  Cybersickness Theories ............................. 5
     1.2.3  Presence ............................................. 6
     1.2.4  Embodiment and Avatar Vision ..................... 7
     1.2.5  Head-Mounted Displays (HMD) and Cybersickness ....... 7
     1.2.6  CAVE and HMD ...................................... 7
  1.3 Technologies Used in VR ...................................... 8
     1.3.1  Head-Mounted Displays (HMDs) ..................... 9
     1.3.2  CAVEs ............................................... 11
     1.3.3  Workbenches ........................................ 14
     1.3.4  Autostereoscopic Displays .......................... 15
     1.3.5  Comparing CAVEs and HMDs ...................... 15
  1.4 Driving Simulation ............................................ 17
     1.4.1  Virtual Reality, Flight Simulation, and Driving
          Simulation ........................................... 18
     1.4.2  Simulation Fidelity .................................. 22
  References ......................................................... 23

**2 Self-motion Perception and Cybersickness** ....................... 31
  2.1 Sensory Organs .............................................. 31
     2.1.1  Visual System ....................................... 31
     2.1.2  Vestibular System ................................... 36
  2.2 Proprioception and Visuo-vestibular Coupling ................ 40

        2.2.1   Optic Flow ........................................... 40
        2.2.2   Vection .............................................. 41
        2.2.3   Vestibulo-ocular Reflex .............................. 44
   2.3   Motion Sickness ......................................... 47
        2.3.1   Sensory Conflict ..................................... 49
        2.3.2   Ecological Theory .................................... 50
        2.3.3   Evolutionary Theory ................................. 51
        2.3.4   Rest Frame .......................................... 51
        2.3.5   Factors Affecting Motion Sickness .................... 52
   2.4   Conclusion .............................................. 55
   References ................................................... 55

**3   Visualization and Motion Systems** ............................. 63
   3.1   Visualization Systems ..................................... 63
        3.1.1   Display Systems ..................................... 63
        3.1.2   A Brief History of HMDs ............................. 75
   3.2   Sensory Excitation Through Motion Platform ................. 77
        3.2.1   Type of Motion Systems and Motion Technologies ........ 77
        3.2.2   Motion Cueing ...................................... 81
   3.3   Walking Systems ......................................... 85
        3.3.1   Unidirectional Treadmills ............................. 85
        3.3.2   Omnidirectional Treadmills ........................... 86
        3.3.3   Gait Devices ........................................ 86
        3.3.4   Walking Spheres ..................................... 87
        3.3.5   Ball Carpets ........................................ 87
        3.3.6   Walking Shoes ...................................... 87
        3.3.7   Mobile Tiles ........................................ 88
        3.3.8   Conclusion .......................................... 88
   References ................................................... 88

**4   Reducing Cybersickness** ..................................... 93
   4.1   Measuring and Predicting VRISE ........................... 93
        4.1.1   Measurements Based on Subjective Features ............. 94
        4.1.2   Measurements Based on Objective Features ............. 99
        4.1.3   Measuring VR Sickness Through Postural Sway
                Analysis ............................................. 100
        4.1.4   Cybersickness Prediction ............................. 102
        4.1.5   Conclusion .......................................... 104
   4.2   Reducing VRISE Through Travel Techniques ................. 104
        4.2.1   Teleportation-Based Techniques ....................... 105
        4.2.2   Motion-Based and Room-Scaled-Based Techniques ....... 106
        4.2.3   Controller-Based Techniques ......................... 107
   4.3   Reducing VRISE by Adapting Existing Travel Techniques ....... 110
        4.3.1   Adaptation of Navigation Parameters ................... 110
        4.3.2   Adaptation Based on Field of View Reduction and Blur .... 110

|  | 4.3.3 | Adaptation Based on Users' Real-Time Physiological State | 111 |
|  | 4.3.4 | Techniques Using Salient Visual References | 112 |
|  | 4.3.5 | Other Adaptation Techniques | 112 |
| 4.4 |  | Reducing VRISE Through Galvanic Stimulation | 112 |
| 4.5 |  | Reducing VRISE Through Auditory Stimulation | 114 |
| 4.6 |  | Best Practices for VRISE Avoidance | 115 |
|  | 4.6.1 | Visuo-Vestibular Coherence in Navigation: Accelerations | 115 |
|  | 4.6.2 | Interactions and Control of Movement | 117 |
|  | 4.6.3 | Field of View | 117 |
|  | 4.6.4 | Latency | 118 |
|  | 4.6.5 | Duration of Exposure | 119 |
|  | 4.6.6 | Independent Visual References | 119 |
|  | 4.6.7 | Binocular Disparity and Depth Cues | 120 |
|  | 4.6.8 | Avatars | 120 |
|  | 4.6.9 | Ecological Setup and Experience | 121 |
|  | References | | 123 |

**5 Applications** ... 133
| 5.1 | Engineering Design and Manufacturing | 133 |
| 5.2 | Simulation for ADAS and AD Development | 136 |
| 5.3 | Vehicle-in-the-Loop Simulation | 136 |
| 5.4 | Architecture and Cultural Heritage Visualization | 138 |
| 5.5 | Videogames | 140 |
| 5.6 | Collaborative Working and Avatars | 141 |
|  | References | 141 |

**6 Conclusion** ... 143
| 6.1 | Virtual Reality and Cybersickness | 143 |
| 6.2 | How to Avoid Cybersickness | 144 |
| 6.3 | Future Trends | 145 |

**Index** ... 147

# Abbreviations

| | |
|---|---|
| AD | Autonomous Driving |
| ADAS | Advanced Driver Assistance Systems |
| AMOLED | Active-Matrix Organic Light-Emitting Diode |
| AR | Augmented Reality |
| BIM | Building Information Modeling |
| CAVE | Cave Automatic Virtual Environment |
| CGI | Computer-Generated Images |
| COG | Center Of Gravity |
| CRT | Cathode-Ray Tube |
| CSDV | Cybersickness Dose Value |
| DIL | Driver In-the-Loop |
| DLP | Digital Light Processing |
| DMD | Digital Micromirror Device |
| DOF | Degree Of Freedom |
| ECG | Electrocardiography |
| EDA | Electrodermal Activity |
| EEG | Electroencephalography |
| EGG | Electrogastrography |
| FHD | Full High Definition |
| FOV | Field Of View |
| GVS | Galvanic Vestibular Stimulation |
| HMD | Head-Mounted Display |
| HMI | Human–Machine Interface |
| HUD | Head-Up Display |
| IPD | Inter-Pupillary Distance |
| LCD | Liquid-Crystal Display |
| LED | Light-Emitting Diode |
| MCA | Motion Cueing Algorithm |
| MISC | MIsery SCale |
| MPC | Model Predictive Control |
| MR | Mixed Reality |
| MSDV | Motion Sickness Dose Value |

| | |
|---|---|
| MSHQ | Motion Sickness History Questionnaire |
| MSSQ | Motion Sickness Susceptibility Questionnaire |
| MTP | Motion To Photon |
| OLED | Organic Light-Emitting Diode |
| SSQ | Simulator Sickness Questionnaire |
| UHD | Ultra High Definition |
| VIL | Vehicle In-the-Loop |
| VIMS | Visually Induced Motion Sickness |
| VIMSSQ | Visually Induced Motion Sickness Susceptibility Questionnaire |
| VMU | Virtual Mock-Up |
| VOR | Vestibulo-Ocular Reflex |
| VR | Virtual Reality |
| VRISE | Virtual Reality Induced Sickness Effects |
| XR | eXtended Reality |

# Chapter 1
# Introduction

**Abstract** Virtual Reality (VR), despite the first developments going back to the 1960s, is witnessing an increasing interest since 2013—the year of the release of the affordable Oculus VR Head-Mounted Displays (HMD). This chapter discusses not only the various ways to define VR, providing an overview and insight but also the caveats of using virtual, augmented, and mixed reality. The recent sanitary conditions have proved to be one of the difficulties that may arise when using VR. Unfortunately, there is another significant factor slowing down the VR helmet introduction in the market. This is a new disappointment after the setback of the Nintendo's Virtual Boy, probably way ahead of its time in the 1990s, due to the generated headaches, linked to a since then well-studied phenomenon, namely, cybersickness. After introducing cybersickness and its main effects, also called VR Induced Sickness Effects (VRISE), a short comparison of its manifestation with HMDs, and other virtual spaces (VR rooms, CAVEs, and VR simulators) are shortly discussed. An introduction to virtual reality systems and the corresponding technologies—described more in detail in Chap. 3—completes this chapter, to provide the first insight into cybersickness.

Virtual reality (VR), despite its first developments from the 1960s, is witnessing a great interest since 2013, when the first affordable VR head-mounted displays (HMD) with associated software development kits, such as the Oculus Rift DK1, were released for the general public. The availability of low-cost VR technologies allowed for a better diffusion of these technologies only in numerous application fields, starting with video games, but also in industry (Berg and Vance 2017), health (Ruthenbeck and Reynolds 2015), construction work (Paes and Irizarry 2018), cultural heritage (Bekele et al. 2018), training (Prasolova-Førland et al. 2017), education (Merchant et al. 2014), and many more.

According to Gartner, who regularly publishes its now well-known hype cycle for new technologies, in 2016, VR passed the end of disillusionment where it has been for

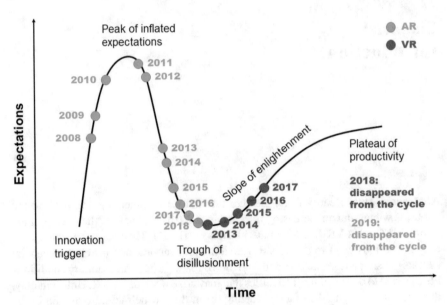

**Fig. 1.1** Evolution of VR and AR on Gartner's hype cycle

several years. In 2017, VR was on the slope of enlightenment, and in 2018, it disappeared from the cycle,[1] leading to progressive development of the market. On the other hand, Augmented Reality (AR) generated high expectations through promising applications, especially in the industry; however, these expectations quickly vanished due to its still low technological maturity. Still, according to Gartner's hype cycle, AR became a mature enough technology as it disappeared from the cycle[2] (Fig. 1.1).

In 2019, several consulting companies estimated the VR market to be about US$11 billion, with a prediction of exponential growth by 2024 (between US$50 and US$88 billion) and a more and more developed content offer.[3]

The development of VR also holds an intensified interest from industry: according to a report from Capgemini released in 2018, about three-fourth of the industrial companies increased their operational profits by more than 10% using VR in their process.[4]

---

[1] Gartner, Hype Cycle for Emerging Technologies, 2018: https://www.gartner.com/doc/3885468?ref=mrktg-srch.

[2] Gartner, 5 Trends Appear on the Gartner Hype Cycle for Emerging Technologies, 2019: https://www.gartner.com/smarterwithgartner/5-trends-appear-on-the-gartner-hype-cycle-for-emerging-technologies-2019/.

[3] Mordor Intelligence, Virtual Reality (VR) Market—Growth, Trends, and Forecast (2020–2025), 2020: https://www.mordorintelligence.com/industry-reports/virtual-reality-market.

[4] Capgemini, Augmented and Virtual Reality in Operations: A guide for investment, 2018: https://www.capgemini.com/research-old/augmented-and-virtual-reality-in-operations/.

# 1.1 Virtual Reality, Augmented Reality, Mixed Reality: Definitions

## 1.1.1 Virtual Reality

Since virtual reality has gathered interest, many definitions were provided, some of them being contradictory, which inevitably leads to high confusion among potential users. For example, many consider that experiencing virtual reality means being immersed in a virtual world or 360° videos, using an HMD, for example.

The origin of the term *Virtual Reality* is not clearly stated. Sources indicate that this term was first used in 1938 by a French writer, Antonin Artaud, who used the term "*réalité virtuelle*" to describe the illusory nature of characters and objects in the theater. The term "virtual reality" was first used in a science-fiction novel, *The Judas Mandala*, in 1982 by Damien Broderick, but did not refer to the current definition of VR. In its current definition, the term was popularized by Jaron Lanier in 1987 and is defined as a computer-generated environment that a user can explore and interact with, solely or along with other users. It is worth noting that though this term was spread in the late 1980s, work on virtual reality was already performed for several decades, but under a different term,—namely, *artificial reality*.

The aim of virtual reality is to allow a user (or several users) a *sensory-motor* activity in a *synthetic world* (Fuchs et al. 2003). Precisely, the specificity of virtual reality is the ability for a user to be fully *immersed* in a virtual environment *and to interact with it* (Sherman and Craig 2003). The most important term here is "interaction", which means that action occurs back and forth between the user and the virtual world. Therefore, we could say that visualizing 360° videos in an HMD is not experiencing virtual reality.

## 1.1.2 Augmented Reality

*Augmented reality* is a term coined by Tom Caudell in 1990 and is defined as a technology that overlays computer-generated images on a view of the *real world*. The user sees the real world, keeping his or her visual references, but this world is "*augmented*" by or combined with a *synthetic world to interact* with. The superimposition can be performed using either devices with embedded cameras (e.g., smartphones and tablet PCs) or glasses.

As in virtual reality, the specificity of augmented reality is to allow interaction with overlaid virtual objects. The primary issue with augmented reality is to track the link between the virtual objects and the real world in real time, whatever the user's position is.

**Reality-virtuality continuum**

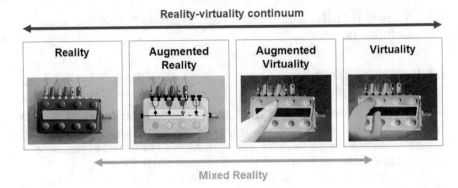

**Fig. 1.2** The reality–virtuality continuum

## 1.1.3 Mixed Reality

*Mixed reality* was introduced in 1994 by Milgram and Kishino (1994) and is defined as a merge of real and virtual worlds that allows users to interact with both real and virtual objects. Mixed reality is not necessarily in either the physical or virtual world but is a composition of physical and virtual reality. The term covers Augmented Reality and Augmented Virtuality, the difference between the two is defined by the "real" or "virtual" predominance of the primarily experienced world.

The reality–virtuality continuum defined by Paul Milgram and Fumio Kishino describes a range between completely real (reality) and completely virtual (virtuality) (Fig. 1.2).

Though this continuum is generally cited to explain the differences between AR, VR, and MR, from a purely logical perspective, the distinction between the different areas is not trivial. For instance, a comparison between Augmented Virtuality and Augmented Reality is often arguable. More controversially, mixed reality which is supposed to encompass Augmented Reality, and Augmented Virtuality is often confused with augmented reality. Typically, the Microsoft HoloLens headset is defined as being an MR display, whereas it is rarely used for Augmented Virtuality and is mostly used as an augmented reality device.

## 1.1.4 What About XR?

Recently, the term *XR* has become trendy. Some use XR for extended reality, which encompasses well beyond mixed reality. Indeed, extended reality is often referred to as both augmented reality and virtual reality, and, sometimes, 360° videos. In this way, XR is not just a technological concept but also defines the usages of these technologies. Indeed, many issues (scientific ones and those related to hardware and software) concerning VR and AR are similar. Therefore, XR is seen as an investigation domain dealing with these technologies.

Nevertheless, with the introduction of various VR and AR devices, some of which usable as VR or AR systems, X is increasingly used as being either Augmented, Virtual, or Mixed.

## 1.2  Cybersickness, VR Sickness, Simulator Sickness, Motion Sickness, and VRISE: Definitions

VR is increasingly gaining popularity, thanks to the recent uptake of relatively cheap VR helmets such as Oculus Rift, HTC Vive, PlayStation VR, and Google Cardboard. However, the long-standing cybersickness issue has not been fixed yet and is likely to be a major obstacle to the mass adoption of VR.

### 1.2.1  Definition

When traveling in a vehicle, passengers can encounter a range of sickness symptoms, from discomfort to nausea through dizziness or vomiting and more (Reason and Brand 1975), which is commonly referred to as car sickness, air sickness, sea sickness, or, generally, vehicle sickness. *Cybersickness* or also called Virtual Reality Induced Sickness Effects (VRISE) and simulator sickness are reported to produce similar sickness effects as motion sickness (Kemeny 2014; Mazloumi Gavgani et al. 2018). Even if the situations that cause it are slightly different, the underlying mechanisms may be explained the same way. Cybersickness is a phenomenon involving nausea and discomfort that can last for hours after experimenting VR applications, linked to the discrepancies of perceived motion between real and virtual worlds.

Cybersickness and simulator sickness were largely studied and described in studies on maneuvers in flight and driving simulators, and they became a well-known and well-described phenomenon following the work of Robert Kennedy in the 1970s.

### 1.2.2  Cybersickness Theories

Three theories, in particular, try to explain cybersickness: sensory conflict theory, ecological theory, and poison theory.

The sensory conflict theory is most popular (Harm 2002), and it suggests that cybersickness is caused by a mismatch between the sensory systems involved in motion perception. Visuo-vestibular conflict is thought to have a prevalent impact.

The ecological theory (Riccio and Stoffregen 1991) states that simulator sickness is caused by a prolonged period of postural instability during travel. This theory also predicts that postural instability precedes sickness (Stoffregen and Smart 1998). Kennedy introduced postural stability measures as early as in 1996 to quantify cybersickness (Kennedy and Stanney 1996).

Finally, the poison theory states that cybersickness symptoms come from an evolutionary mechanism that occurs when one is experiencing sensory hallucinations (Treisman 1977). This mechanism aims at ejecting ingested toxic substances, thus explaining nausea and vomiting. This theory remains controversial as the time needed for a toxin to affect the vestibular mechanisms seems too long for vomiting to be effective (Harm 2002).

A piece of research achieves VRISE reduction in very specific conditions (Kemeny et al. 2015; Fernandes and Feiner 2016; Wienrich et al. 2018)—hence the need to be careful in the development of VR experiences, especially when designing navigation techniques.

More detailed descriptions of cybersickness theories and proposals to reduce them are given in Chaps. 2 and 4, respectively.

### 1.2.3 Presence

If cybersickness is a critical issue when it comes to taking advantage of immersive technologies; another essential factor to consider to maximize the quality of immersive experience is the sense of presence, which is defined as the sense of "being there"—physically present in the virtual environment (Sheridan 1992; Slater and Wilbur 1997). Highly present people should act in a virtual environment as if they were in a real one and should remember the experience more as a place they visited than as pictures they saw (Slater and Wilbur 1997). According to Slater (Slater 2009), this illusion of being in a place—called Place Illusion—should be complemented by the illusion—called Plausibility Illusion—that what is happening in the virtual environment is really happening, so that people who experience it behave realistically.

Past studies tried to establish a relation between presence and cybersickness (see (Weech et al. 2019) for a survey). This relation may not be straightforward as indicated by past research, which described either a positive correlation or a negative or no correlation. However, from what Weech et al. (2019) argue, it is likely that cybersickness and presence are negatively correlated, which might be explained by several factors, such as display conditions (stereoscopy, field of view), or navigation control.

### 1.2.4    Embodiment and Avatar Vision

When wearing a head-mounted display, people may become shielded from reality. This may affect spatial orientation, which, in turn, can influence motion sickness (Kennedy et al. 2010). A way to better immerse users is by using avatars for the visualization of both their own body and those of other participants interacting in collaborative working or gaming in the same virtual world. An avatar is a representation of a user's body in the virtual world through the visualization of his or her body and its interactions with the direct environment. This representation renders the body's position, movement, and gestures. In many applications involving collaboration in which users do not have a body's representation, avatars are proposed progressively.

The vision of a virtual body and the sense of embodiment (i.e., the capacity to own, control, and be inside an avatar's body)—in particular, its role in improving users' immersive experience—have been widely studied. Kilteni et al. (2012) demonstrated that the sense of embodiment is crucial for presence: still, the link between embodiment and cybersickness is not wholly clear. Some research indicates that adding, for example, a virtual nose or an avatar can alleviate cybersickness effects (Hecht 2016).

### 1.2.5    Head-Mounted Displays (HMD) and Cybersickness

If VR helmets generate cybersickness—the more immersive they are, the more cybersickness generator they are—AR helmets rarely produce sickness effects, though their tendency to do so depends on helmet characteristics, which is linked to their visual rendering qualities, namely, to their level of immersivity. Often, their visual Field Of View (FOV) is limited, as they may be designed to complete real-world perception with Computer-Generated Images (CGI), thus affecting the perception of the observer less than with VR helmets. The presence of real-world visual references keeps the observers in their usual stability conditions, thus remarkably reducing sickness effects (see Sect. 4.3.4).

### 1.2.6    CAVE and HMD

There is a growing debate about the respective advantages of Cave Automatic Virtual Environment (CAVE) or immersive rooms and HMDs with more and more users adopting HMD technology. It can be surprising to observe the renewal of this trend, knowing that HMD was already introduced in 1968. Yet, at the time, it lacked computer-generated images, and it has experienced several severe setbacks since then (Oliver 2018).

Indeed, CAVEs, though much more expensive, allow keeping both the user's body and other tangible objects the user interacts with visible, which makes it possible to share the experience with up to six users with recent techniques (Chapman 2018) who are equally immersed (having their head tracked, having their own observation axis and stereoscopic view, and seeing the same virtual scene). This may also let the user(s) combine the virtual scene with real objects, such as a Virtual Mock-Up (VMU), that they can touch and feel. Finally, another significant advantage is that the users seeing real objects (not only their own body, but also the apparent structure of the CAVE though easily and quickly integrated by the viewer during immersion) keep seeing stable external references, which reduces cybersickness, if other VRISE parameters, such as image lag, incomplete or unstable head tracking, and subsequent flawed motion parallax, do not ruin these benefits. Unfortunately, the lack of sufficiently high-frequency image rendering and low transport delays (the lag between actions and corresponding rendered images) may severely limit this potential advantage (Colombet et al. 2016).

Another consideration is the massive arrival of robust AR HMDs with high-resolution and high-frequency image rendering capabilities and optical (Vovk et al. 2018) or video (Rolland et al. 1995; Combe et al. 2008a) see-through technology. Optical see-through HMDs get most of the advantages of CAVEs for reduced cyber-sickness at significantly more affordable prices and installation constraints, though wearing the helmets is still intrusive and may produce eye fatigue and sickness effects (Hua 2017; Iskander et al. 2018). Video see-through helmets bring now increased computational capabilities by integrating a broad set of world scanning and integra-tion techniques. However, the collocation of camera-viewed images in correspon-dence to the eye position[5] and the integration of different image sources are still subjects of intensive research and VR technology development (Kruijff et al. 2010).

## 1.3 Technologies Used in VR

Since the first developments of VR in the 1960s (Sutherland 1968), several visu-alization devices were built and proposed. The main ones are the HMDs and the CAVEs.

---

[5]The collocation of the viewer eyes and a camera for video see-through helmets is a challenging difficulty as the captured images are not instantaneously available (the camera cannot be placed in front of the eyes). New emerging techniques may capture and compensate the resulting gap, but again with the introduction of additional lag in the already often insufficiently reduced transport delay.

## 1.3.1 Head-Mounted Displays (HMDs)

The first HMD for Virtual and Augmented Reality was built in 1968; back then, it could display wired frame images only (Sutherland 1968). The last decade has seen the development of affordable head-mounted displays, such as the HTC Vive or the Oculus Rift, which currently represent flagship products among all the helmets available in the market.

VR helmets are usually characterized by one or more screen(s) placed in front of the user's eyes. This display shows two images, one for each eye. Because of the distance between the eyes and the screen and the size of the screen, Fresnel lenses are usually mounted on the screen to get a 1:1 scale. Today, images are rendered at an around 90 Hz frequency and up to 110 Hz for the latest technologies, with at least 2.5 K resolution per eye for the most common headsets. High-resolution displays (4 K, or even 8 K) have been progressively introduced in the market.

A tracking system, usually based on infrared cameras, allows users to be accurately tracked in a specific area defined by the users. Several HMDs in the market allow a field of view of around 110°. Recent models can achieve a 200° field of view. This aspect is not negligible, as the field of view has a significant role in the occurrence of cybersickness (Lin et al. 2002).

In most HMDs, the distance of accommodation is fixed and depends on the geometrical and optical design of the helmet. Focus cues are thus not rendered—namely, the accommodation of the observer's eyes is remaining constant whatever the distance to the observed virtual object is. In contrast to real conditions, focus cues and vergence (rotation of the eyes according to the distance of the observed object) are then decoupled, especially when the viewed objects are close, inducing a strong accommodation, which leads to a vergence-accommodation conflict (Fig. 1.3). This conflict also exists in CAVEs, even though the observer can modify the distance to the screens while walking, and it can lead to symptoms varying from discomfort and fatigue to nausea, besides pathologies in the developing visual system of children (Rushton and Riddell 1999). As correct or nearly correct focus cues affect perceived depth (Watt et al. 2005; Held et al. 2012), a "light field stereoscope" has been developed by Huang et al. (2015). Specifically, this stereoscope is a wearable VR display in which a light field instead of traditional 2D images is presented to each eye, allowing the eyes to freely focus within the scene (see Chap. 3, Sect. 3.1).

Another important issue in VR technology is the transport delay—the delay between the action and the corresponding rendering cues—which depends on several factors, such as the image frequency rate, motion rendering, and the way the user's actions are captured (Kemeny 2001). Cybersickness is likely to occur as this delay increases (LaViola 2000). Even small delays can induce nausea since the system responsible for eye fixations works very quickly (around 20 ms) (Berthoz 2000). With the progress in computational power and electronics, recent virtual reality devices present low-latency characteristics (around 15 ms). Hence, we would imagine latency to be less critical. However, not considering this parameter would be wrong, as VR applications become more and more power-consuming with the possible adjunction

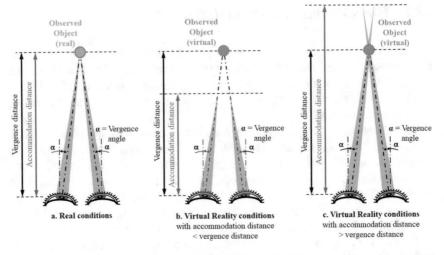

**Fig. 1.3** Illustration of the vergence-accommodation conflict. In real conditions (**a**), vergence distance and accommodation distance are identical. In Virtual Reality, the vergence distance induced by stereoscopy generally differs from the accommodation distance (either being smaller in **b** or greater in **c**)

of VR device add-ons such as trackers and dynamical platforms. Furthermore, we should not forget that any physical device will always have a latency.

The luminosity of the integrated display system may also have a strong impact not only on the perceived image quality but also on distance perception. Previous studies indicate that the overall luminosity in the observed real-world environment may influence distance perception (Coello and Grealy 1997), which may be the cause of impaired distance and thus scale perception in VR systems, especially in HMDs, where the displayed luminosity is significatively lower than in real-world scenes. Furthermore, in the case of video see-through HMDs, impaired perception may be the result of the differences in providing real-world stereoscopic images captured by the camera and virtual world images computed by the image rendering system (Hale and Stanney 2006). However, major differences may be observed between optical see-through and video see-through headsets, as composing images of different sources may induce perceptual differences, for example, in distance or size perception (Combe et al. 2008b). Though optical see-through headsets have their drawbacks, the luminosity and color dynamics of virtual images is significantly lower than that of real images. Microsoft's HoloLens or comparable AR headsets are equipped with state-of-the-art display systems, limiting these undesirable effects, even if Microsoft recommends only indoor usage.[6] Dynamic calibration for a large range of illumination conditions is still an ongoing challenge for deploying AR systems in all lighting conditions.

---

[6]Microsoft, Environment considerations for HoloLens, 2019: https://docs.microsoft.com/en-us/hol olens/hololens-environment-considerations.

## *1.3.2 CAVEs*

A Cave Automatic Virtual Environment (CAVE) is an immersive display consisting of several large screens (often around 3 m wide), usually assembled in a squared shape. Rectangular or circular CAVEs also exist. Unlike HMDs, images are displayed to users by video projectors like in 3D theaters. Users wear special glasses that make it possible to render stereoscopy appropriately. Several technologies exist to render stereoscopy either passively or actively (see Chap. 3, Sect. 3.1.1). In passive stereoscopy, the two images for both eyes are displayed at the same time, as each image is projected by one video projector. Images are displayed for the two eyes separately, thanks to the use of polarization (Ostnes et al. 2004) or spectral filtering technologies based on interference filters, such as INFITEC (Schmieder et al. 2017), masking one of the two images for each eye. Passive stereoscopy requires filters for the projectors as well as for the glasses that the observer must wear. Stereoscopy is achieved by the glasses that combine the polarized or filtered images. In active stereoscopy, the glasses shut each eye alternatively at a high frequency by means of liquid crystals included in the glasses (Ostnes et al. 2004). For multiuser observation, several of these techniques can be combined (Chen et al. 2015). However, at present, a half dozen independent users can view stereoscopic images with an independent observation axis, each having their tracking device, which provides correct motion parallax cues (Chapman 2018).

As for HMDs, a tracking system is included in CAVEs that allows users to be tracked within the area of the CAVEs. Infrared cameras are installed at each corner of the CAVE, and patterns of light-reflective balls are mounted on the glasses.

The first CAVE installations arrived in the early 1990s (Cruz-Neira et al. 1992). In France, the first CAVE was installed at Institut Image of Arts et Métiers in Chalon-sur-Saône (France) in 2001, and it consisted of a four-sided CAVE that was reconfigurable for the purpose of the applications. It was updated in 2018 to a five-sided 4 K-resolution CAVE, called the BlueLemon, enabling two viewpoints at the same time for collaborative tasks (Fig. 1.4).

The CAVE system is used in several companies as a tool for applications such as collaborative project design review or simulations. An example is provided by the French car manufacturer Renault where the high-performance CAVE—a 70 M 3D pixel five-sided 4 K technology-based CAVE—is used by designers, ergonomists, and vehicle architects to design new vehicles (Fig. 1.5). To prevent the used high luminosity from causing inter-wall interferences, 3 acrylic walls with a special gain are used, providing a high contrast quality.

Each CAVE system is usually unique in its design and characteristics, though now some suppliers, such as Barco, offer off-the-shelf transportable configurations.[7] Some of them present particular settings.

The C6 (Virtual Reality Applications—Iowa State University, USA) is a 10 × 10 × 10 ft (3.05 × 3.05 × 3.05 m) CAVE, and has six sides and a 100 M pixel resolution (Oliver 2018) (Fig. 1.6).

---

[7]Barco, Transportable cave: https://www.barco.com/en/product/transportable-cave.

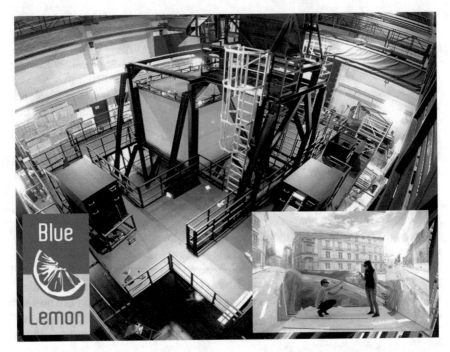

**Fig. 1.4** The BlueLemon at Institut Image of Arts et Métiers (France)

The Tore (University of Lille, France) is a 4 × 8 × 4 m flattened semispherical-shaped CAVE; thanks to its shape, there is no visible edge, which can enhance the immersion level.[8]

Immersia (IRISA, Rennes, France) is a four-sided CAVE with large dimensions (9.6 × 3.1 × 3 m) and a 46 M pixel resolution, allowing real walking.[9]

The CAVE2 (EVL, University of Illinois at Chicago, USA) is a large-scale system composed of 72 3D LCD panels for a total resolution of 37 M 3D pixels. The screens are arranged in a circular shape allowing a 320° field of view.[10]

Most CAVE systems are usually dedicated to applications that do not require much movement, such as design review sessions. However, there exists a trend of large CAVE systems where people can walk for real. These CAVEs are often used for pedestrian simulation applications such as street crossing. Examples are the one at the University of Gustave Eiffel (ex-IFSTTAR, France) (Cavallo et al. 2016) (Fig. 1.7 left), the HIKER lab at the University of Leeds (UK) (Sadraei et al. 2020) (Fig. 1.7 right), or the one at the University of Iowa (USA) (Rahimian et al. 2015).

---

[8] AV Magazine, University of Lille installs world-first CAVE design, 2018: https://www.avinteractive.com/news/virtual-augmented-mixed/university-lille-installs-world-first-cave-design-21-06-2018/.

[9] IRISA, Immersia: http://www.irisa.fr/immersia/technical-description/.

[10] EVL, CAVE2: Next-Generation Virtual-Reality and Visualization Hybrid Environment for Immersive Simulation and Information Analysis: https://www.evl.uic.edu/entry.php?id=2016.

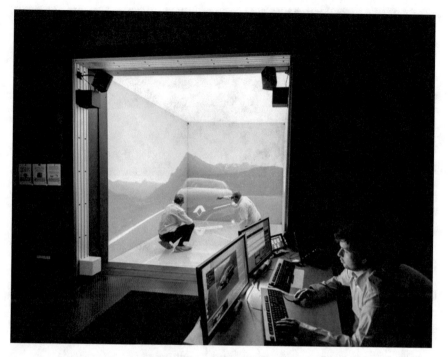

**Fig. 1.5** Renault's 70 M 3D pixels 5-sided high-performance CAVE (France)

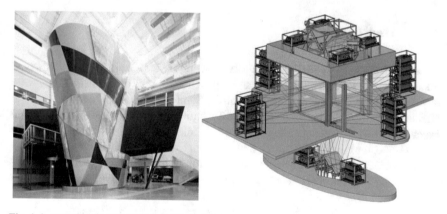

**Fig. 1.6** VRAC's C6 CAVE (Oliver 2018) (USA)

The automotive industry was an early adopter with General Motors,[11] and most of the major carmakers today own one or several CAVEs, though many turn to

[11] WardsAuto, GM Uses Virtual World to Perfect Future Vehicles, 2016: https://www.wardsauto.com/industry/gm-uses-virtual-world-perfect-future-vehicles.

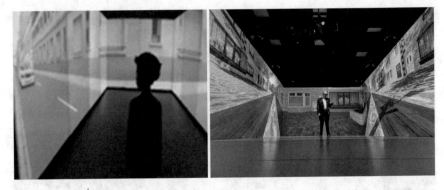

**Fig. 1.7** Left: University Gustave Eiffel's street-crossing simulator (France). Right: HIKER lab at the University of Leeds (UK)

HMDs[12] like companies from the aerospace industry,[13] strong HMD users from the beginnings.

Finally, it is a meaningful sign that more and more installations, such as those of the University of Gustave Eiffel and the University of Leeds, combine driving simulators and CAVEs. Furthermore, many recent driving simulators use CAVE-like visual environments or HMDs (Lyga et al. 2020). The convergence of driving simulators and VR or AR systems, sharing some of the drawbacks of virtual environments, namely, motion and cybersickness, can thus be witnessed (Kemeny 2014).

### 1.3.3  Workbenches

Workbenches are large display monitors allowing several users to view displayed images and interact with them. They can be tilted horizontally or vertically. They were developed at the Naval Research Laboratory, Stanford University, and the German National Research Center for Information Technology (GMD) in 1994 (Krueger and Froehlich 1994; Krueger et al. 1995) and were called Responsive Workbenches. The original version consisted of only one horizontal monitor on which stereoscopic images were projected by a projector-and-mirror system. Fakespace, Inc. marketed the Responsive Workbench as the Immersive Workbench in 1996, and its viewing surface was $100 \times 75$ in ($254 \times 191$ cm). Monitors can be combined—for instance, one horizontal and the other vertical—to form a larger interaction space.

As in CAVE systems, the user's head can be tracked to fit the images to the viewpoint. When several users are present around the workbench, the viewpoint, however,

---

[12]Audi MediaCenter, Audi tests "virtual reality holodeck" for faster product development, 2018: https://www.audi-mediacenter.com/en/press-releases/audi-tests-virtual-reality-holodeck-for-faster-product-development-9873.

[13]VRWorldTech, Airbus partners with Microsoft for HoloLens 2 solutions, 2019: https://vrworldtech.com/2019/06/18/airbus-partners-with-microsoft-for-hololens-2-solutions/.

is adapted to only one user, which may lead to incorrect perspective and complicated interaction with the virtual content. To improve collaborative work, a dual viewpoint workbench was presented by Fakespace in 1997 that allowed two users to have their own stereoscopic viewpoints from the same projection system (Agrawala et al. 1997). Workbenches are usually considered as semi-immersive, as the size of the displays does not allow full immersion as in CAVE systems, for instance, and they are used in collaborative work, such as engineering design, architectural design, scientific visualization, and medicine (Fröhlich et al. 1995; Rosenblum et al. 1997; Weyrich and Drews 1999; Kuester et al. 2000). Workbenches have multiple advantages, in addition to keeping external visual references, thus reducing VRISE; they also allow the integration of different perceptual modalities, namely, visual and haptic, helping the human brains to get a robust perception of user's actions (Ernst and Bülthoff 2004). Workbenches can also be used as an AR platform to visualize virtual mockup assembly processes for manufacturing design.[14]

### 1.3.4 Autostereoscopic Displays

A last category of technologies relies on autostereoscopy, which is based on lenticular lenses or parallax barriers (Dodgson 2005; Järvenpää and Salmimaa 2008). The left and right images are cut into strips. The images are then interlaced to form interlaced strips. The display renders a stereoscopic image through a lenticular lens made of half-cylindrical lenses of the size of one interlaced left-right strip; each interlaced strip is displayed through each lens. The human eyes perceive each strip accordingly, and the brain fusions the left and right strips to build an image including depth.

The main advantage of autostereoscopic displays is that they do not require to wear glasses as in CAVEs. The Nintendo 3DS game console uses this principle to allow for stereoscopic images without glasses. Another interesting feature is the enabling of multi-view projection by rendering one image per viewpoint, thanks to multiple video projectors, as proposed by Holografika. This feature can be used in collaborative applications (see Chap. 3, Sect. 3.1.1).

### 1.3.5 Comparing CAVEs and HMDs

A CAVE and an HMD are very different devices though they both allow one to be immersed in a 3D environment. Differences can be detailed as follows.

---

[14]HoloMake: https://vimeo.com/262513599.

### 1.3.5.1   Cybersickness

CAVE systems may induce less cybersickness than HMDs, as reported by several studies (Polcar and Horejsi 2013). Previous research on the impact of body vision on postural stability (Vaillant et al. 2004; Maria Galeazzi et al. 2006) suggests that one of the reasons for experiencing VRISE could be the lack of own-body visions. This could explain why in CAVEs, where the observer's body and nearby objects are seen, thus providing external visual references and better postural stability, users experience less cybersickness effects. This is still a subject of ongoing research, and one can observe similar simulation sickness effect comparison results between CAVEs and immersive VR helmets in some comparable situations, too (Colombet et al. 2016; Kemeny et al. 2017). Hence, Augmented Reality helmets provide better conditions for applications without cybersickness effects.

### 1.3.5.2   Stereoscopy

In a CAVE, images are displayed through video projectors, and stereoscopic visualization of virtual environments is enabled through glasses. The user's head moves relative to the physical screens; hence, the focus that is made on the screen is always changing. In an HMD, images are displayed through screens placed in front of the user's eyes, and stereoscopy is achieved through lenses. Because the HMD is worn by the user, the distance between the screen and the eyes is constant and very small (usually less than 20 cm, though the accommodation distance is bigger, thanks to the lenses). This difference in image viewing distance raises a well-known effect called the accommodation-vergence conflict that generates visual fatigue (Hoffman et al. 2008). Recent studies suggest that CAVEs are better suited for correct proximal depth perception, while HMDs are to be preferred for longer distances (Ghinea et al. 2018), as increased underestimation was observed for positive parallax conditions and slight overestimation for negative and zero parallax conditions (Bruder et al. 2016).

Motion parallax is one of the most crucial cues in the depth perception. To provide it, we need to use head trackers, which unfortunately may introduce lags (transport delay) in providing the images to display, thus inducing VRISE. The inter-pupillary distance (IPD) is another factor that is of major importance in stereoscopic rendering: inaccurate adjustment of images with the user's IPD may bias perception (including distance and depth), which may also induce cybersickness (Rebenitsch and Owen 2016).

### 1.3.5.3   Distance Perception

It is widely acknowledged that size and distance perception in virtual reality seems modified. In particular, the literature indicates that distances are generally underestimated in virtual environments of about 50% when compared to the real world (Renner et al. 2013). Past work indicates that HMDs provide better distance perception for large distances (>8 m), while CAVEs provide better perception for close distances (Ghinea et al. 2018). However, differences in performance regarding distance perception may be explained by a combination of other factors, such as the use of unnatural interfaces, the graphics quality of a virtual environment (though the latter seems not to have any significant impact on distance perception (Thompson et al. 2004)), the virtual camera tuning relative to users' inter-pupillary distance, the parallax, the distance to the screen (Bruder et al. 2016), or even users' cognitive profile (Boustila et al. 2015).

### 1.3.5.4 Body Ownership

In an HMD, the user is shielded from the real world, which ensures a high level of immersion. However, the user no longer sees his/her body, leading to rely on proprioceptive cues only. Conversely, in a CAVE, the user still sees it.

### 1.3.5.5 Available Workspace

A CAVE is usually limited in physical space by the size of the screens (e.g., 3 m by 3 m). Therefore, physical movements are limited within this space. In an HMD, as it is worn, theoretically, the available workspace corresponds to the area of the virtual environment. Although the latest devices are wireless, in practice, the physical workspace is limited by the wires attached to the HMD and by the tracking system.

### 1.3.5.6 Price

Recently released HMDs are sold at less than US$1,000. Bundled with a PC with appropriate specifications (VR-ready graphic card), a full HMD kit costs around US$3,000. Standalone versions also exist for less than US$500. A CAVE is way more expensive. Indeed, there are no on-the-shelf CAVEs in the market. All systems are made upon request to meet specific requirements. High-end systems can rise to US$1 million, while low-cost systems may only cost US$50,000, depending on the screen size, material, video projectors, structure, tracking system, computers, among others.

## 1.4 Driving Simulation

Cybersickness is not only experienced in virtual reality, but was also reported and studied early in aeronautical research on flight and helicopter simulators (Kennedy and Frank 1985; Groen et al. 2007). However, there exists another vast simulation field where motion sickness is often experienced and probably with even more widely perceived societal consequences: the automotive industry (Kemeny and Panerai 2003).

### 1.4.1  Virtual Reality, Flight Simulation, and Driving Simulation

Flight simulators, using computer-generated imagery since the 1980s (Yan 1985), were probably the first VR systems with users experiencing cybersickness. Sickness effects were measured, and Robert Kennedy (Kennedy et al. 1993) soon built the now well-known Simulator Sickness Questionnaire (SSQ)—a sickness survey with various recent versions. The original version was foreseen from the very beginning to measure cybersickness in VR (Kennedy et al. 1992), and, subsequently, various modified versions were proposed, such as the MIsery SCale (MISC) (Bos et al. 2005) (see Chap. 4, Sect. 4.1).

Recently, several studies have emphasized the future impact of motion sickness for autonomous vehicles, as a large part of autonomous vehicle users will experience motion sickness (Diels 2014; Sivak and Schoettle 2015; Diels et al. 2016; Diels and Bos 2016; Iskander et al. 2019). Subsequently, researchers and industries may propose motion or virtual reality systems to correct the undesirable effects of motion occurring when the subject is transported (Sawabe et al. 2016; Oliver 2018) without sufficient information. This may help the user anticipate vehicle motion or accept and trust autonomous vehicles (Wintersberger et al. 2019).

#### 1.4.1.1  Driving Simulation for Autonomous Vehicles

Driving simulation is widely used to study and validate these tools and, traditionally, for training or engineering design for Human Machine Interfaces (HMIs) or Advanced Driver Assistance Systems (ADAS) (Reymond and Kemeny 2000; Kemeny and Panerai 2003; Strobl and Huesmann 2004; Bertollini et al. 2010; Langlois 2013). The recent advent of autonomous vehicle development will only increase the necessity of using driving simulation to guarantee that the driver perceives and correctly uses vehicle maneuvers, in particular, when switching from autonomous to manual mode (Merat et al. 2014; Dogan et al. 2017; Zhang et al. 2019). Autonomous vehicle validation will not only be viable through only field tests due to road and driver safety reasons but also because of the huge amount of driving scenarios to be tested and validated (Kalra and Paddock 2016; Sovani 2017; Colmard 2018). Unfortunately, driving simulation is subject to motion and cybersickness (Kemeny and Panerai 2003; Kemeny 2014).

### 1.4.1.2  Driving Simulation and Its Links with Virtual Reality

Driving simulation and virtual reality are closely linked, and both technologies started to be developed roughly in the same period—the 1960s and 1970s, respectively. Sutherland developed the first virtual reality head-mounted display in 1968 (Sutherland 1968) even though only with wireframe images; furthermore, the helmets were not interactive. In the same period, the first real-time CGI systems were developed by General Electric, yet only displaying a couple of dozen non-textured polygons. Doron Electronics, founded in 1970, became the first company to develop and produce complete driving simulation systems (Allen et al. 2011), though, at the time only with video visual display of the driving environment. Finally, driving simulator systems benefited from CGI and the use of motion platforms in the 1970s at VTI (Swedish National Road and Transport Research Institute). The first full-scale motion-based driving simulator was released between 1977 and 1984. Daimler released one with 6 degrees of freedom (DOF) in the late 1980s, which was entirely rebuilt in the 1990s with an enhanced high-performance linear actuator, thus with a 7 DOF motion platform (Nordmark 1976; Drosdol et al. 1985; Käding and Hoffmeyer 1995; Nordmark et al. 2004).

From the very early development period, the driving simulation community also expressed a keen interest in virtual reality technologies, and many simulators were integrated with HMDs. Examples are n-Vision at Volvo (Burns and Saluäär 1999a), ProView VL50 and SEOS at Renault (Coates et al. 2002; Fuchs 2017), a robot-based cybermotion simulator with Sensics XSight (Grabe et al. 2010), and more recently Volkswagen (Hartfiel and Stark 2019). CAVE-like display system- based driving simulators were also released at Renault (Kemeny 2014), and at Porsche (Baumgartner et al. 2019), among others.

### 1.4.1.3  Driving Simulator Sickness

It is then easily understandable that, until recently, many motion and cybersickness studies were initiated using driving simulators. Furthermore, driving simulation and virtual reality share the same or similar difficulties in rendering the movements of the observer in the virtual environments as both of them use Computer-Generated Imagery (CGI) and interactions with sensory feedback and provide physical and mental immersion (Sherman and Craig 2003). However, driving simulation relates to vehicle driving and thus usually implies perception and control of self-motion at a higher range of velocities than in virtual reality where locomotion is often reduced to walking in a virtual environment.

Although drivers are less sensitive to its effects than passengers (Dong and Stoffregen 2010), a significant factor in VRISE is the transport delay between the driver actions and its effects on the rendered perceivable motion (Uliano et al. 1986; Moss et al. 2011; Kemeny et al. 2015). Likewise, although driving is reported in many papers as mostly a visual-dominant task (Sivak 1996), it is also well-established that

other sensory information, such as those provided by the vestibular and proprioceptive channels, contributes to the perception and control of self-motion significantly
(Ritchie et al. 1968).

Many consider as a landmark work on perception for automobile driving the
research carried out in 1938 by Gibson, who proposed a theory defining a "terrain
or field of space" for the driver and considered the car as a tool of locomotion and
the driver as aiming to drive in the middle of a "field of safe travel" (Gibson and
Crooks 1938). The visual perception of space, described by Gibson in 1950, is based
on visual depth, distance, and orientation stimuli.

However, it is not clear whether the same strategies used for natural locomotion
(walking) apply to driving situations where displacements occur at higher velocities.
An interesting point of view on these controversial issues was provided by experiments performed in driving simulators (Rushton and Salvucci 2001; Rushton 2004).
However, Gibson's original theory also included a definition of the perceptual field
of the car itself, rendering kinesthetic and tactile cues to the driver. These ideas were
applied to driving simulation from the early 1980s (Nordmark et al. 1984; Drosdol
et al. 1985; Reymond et al. 2001), and, since then, many simulator experiments have
been carried out for vehicle design (Burns and Saluäär 1999a; Boer 2000; Panerai
et al. 2001), driver behavior, and perception studies (Wierwille et al. 1983; Cavallo
et al. 2001).

### 1.4.1.4    Visual Cues in Driving Simulation

Driving simulators provide many yet not all the relevant visual cues that are present
when driving in the real world. Optic flow, resulting from the continuous movement
of the textured images of all objects in the scene, is present. However, binocular
cues, as well as motion parallax due to the observer's head movement, are often
absent in simulators, though recently a few studies were carried out on their roles
in driving simulation (Schmieder et al. 2017; Perroud et al. 2019). Furthermore, an
increasing number of driving simulators are integrating stereoscopic display systems
(Schmieder et al. 2017; Hartfiel and Stark 2019; Baumgartner et al. 2019).

Depth perception is based upon several visual cues (Cutting and Vishton 1995).
The most well-known ones are binocular, such as vergence, the angle between the
observation axes and disparity, and the difference between the images of the same
object seen by the two eyes (Howard and Rogers 1995). Another depth cue, often
mentioned as crucial and potentially in conflict with vergence cue in a virtual reality
system, is a monocular cue called accommodation.

### 1.4.1.5    Motion Parallax

Nevertheless, motion parallax (see Fig. 1.8) remains a particularly strong monocular
cue. Specifically, it is generally recognized as an independent cue for the perception
of relative distances (Rogers and Graham 1979) that provides robust estimates of

**Fig. 1.8** Illustration of motion parallax. The closer the object, the greater its displacement on the retina during a relative head movement

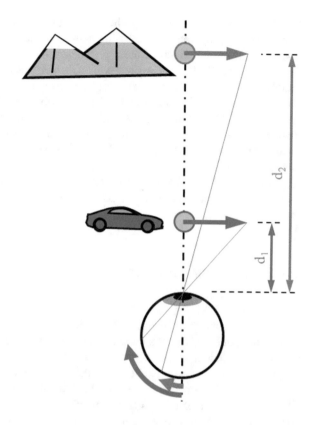

absolute egocentric distances when combined with extraretinal information about the observer's self-motion. Nawrot (2003) demonstrated that eye movements can provide sufficient extraretinal information for efficient integration of motion parallax for depth perception. Furthermore, Panerai et al. (2002) indicated that the central nervous system is able to combine these types of information to account for head movements, even when they are small. This finding suggests that the integration of these two cues is also likely to be effective for natural head movements, such as those occurring during ordinary driving.

Unfortunately, though some recent experiments report motion parallax as provided thanks to head trackers, their role in driving simulation has not been confirmed yet (Perroud et al. 2020), probably because sufficiently low transport delays are difficult to guarantee when computer-generated image frequency is rarely less than 60 Hz. Indeed, the perception of depth from motion parallax occurs with brief stimulus presentations (30 ms), and significantly higher latencies may disrupt depth-discrimination (Nawrot and Stroyan 2012).

Under natural conditions, visual depth cues are redundant in eliciting a robust perception of 3D space. However, in a driving simulator, the number of depth cues might be reduced, and the various display parameters (e.g., image resolution, frequency, and field of view) may alter temporal and spatial distance perception.

Finally, motion cues might be either missing or partially or poorly synchronized with visual information. An increasing number of studies were published in the last two decades on the effects of these parameters on either driving simulator fidelity (Jamson 2000, 2001) or driver behavior (Chatziastros et al. 1999; Colombet et al. 2008), as well as on the comparison of perception in simulators with real driving (Wierwille et al. 1983; Burns and Saluäär 1999b; Boer 2000; Hallvig et al. 2013; Helland et al. 2013). Furthermore, in monoscopic driving simulators, it was observed that drivers may underestimate distances (to a leading vehicle) when compared to driving on a real road (Panerai et al. 2001). However, even if systematic performance analysis of new motion cueing algorithms for driving simulators is now available (Ellensohn et al. 2019; van Leeuwen et al. 2019; Ronellenfitsch et al. 2019), the precise role of motion parallax for distance perception in driving simulation has not been confirmed yet.

### 1.4.2   Simulation Fidelity

The validity of driving simulation experiments is a crucial issue not sufficiently studied yet (Kemeny and Panerai 2003; Helman and Reed 2015; Perroud et al. 2019). Absolute validity of driver simulation, which entails that the driven vehicle's cinematics and behavior are perceived in the same way as in the real world, is not always required for human factor studies; only the assessment of the studied man–machine interface or traffic situation is needed, which requires the relative validity of the simulated driver-vehicle situations (Kemeny 2009). However, the correct perception of speed and acceleration is essential for Advanced Driver Assistance Systems (ADAS) experiments, as vehicle behavior must be simulated correctly. Furthermore, it determines whether the correct mental workload is an issue relative to real immersion, as driver attention is depending on it (Barthou et al. 2010).

Driving simulation studies often require a careful analysis of the complete set of perceptual variables used by the driver. For example, the correct perception of "time headway"—the time interval between two vehicles following one another—is crucial both in studies analyzing driver behavior when using adaptive cruise-control systems that regulate inter-vehicle distance and in autonomous vehicle testing.

The kind of display equipment used can also affect simulation fidelity. For example, a widely cited experiment that involved displaying computer-generated images of the road environment on a computer monitor suggested that drivers' speed perception is significantly reduced in foggy conditions (Snowden et al. 1998), which may influence driver behavior and explain traffic accident statistics in the presence of fog. However, other studies indicate that a too limited fog model for image rendering or a limited field of view induces a poor perception of speed by the driver (Jamson 2000; Pretto and Chatziastros 2006; Pretto et al. 2012). Hence, conclusions derived from computer-based simulations might be insufficient and not validated in real-world experiments (Cavallo 2002). Furthermore, a reduced field of view does not allow to provide sufficient visual information in urban areas when turning—one of the most critical situations for VRISE (Colombet et al. 2016).

Another visual cue, angular declination—the viewing angle between the horizon and a point of the ground plane—was shown to be a strong determinant of perceived distance (Panerai et al. 2001). Interestingly, the Oculus best practices guide (Yao et al. 2014) is citing "looking down" as a factor impacting rendering, realism, or inducing VRISE (Loomis 2001; Ooi et al. 2001). Modification in angular declination may impact perceived distance.

Furthermore, as Gibson pointed out, and as will be discussed in more detail in Chap. 2, kinesthetic cues also strongly influence the perception of speed (Gibson and Crooks 1938; Wierwille et al. 1983). To simulate vestibular stimuli, accelerations to be perceived by the driver can be rendered by the real-time generation of simulator cockpit motion, following appropriate vehicle dynamics. As discussed in Chap. 3, motion cueing is the subject of intense ongoing research, and various motion systems are proposed for affordable to high-performance driving simulators (Colombet et al. 2008; Zeeb 2010; Venrooij et al. 2015; Bruschetta et al. 2017; Romano et al. 2019).

# References

Agrawala M, Beers AC, McDowall I, Fröhlich B, Bolas M, Hanrahan P (1997) The two-user Responsive Workbench: support for collaboration through individual views of a shared space. In: Proceedings of the 24th annual conference on Computer graphics and interactive techniques. ACM Press/Addison-Wesley Publishing Co., USA, pp 327–332

Allen RW, Rosenthal TJ, Cook ML (2011) A short history of driving simulation. In: Hand-book of driving simulation for engineering, medicine and psychology. CRC Press. Taylor and Francis Group, LLC

Barthou A, Kemeny A, Reymond G, Mérienne F, Berthoz A (2010) Driver trust and reliance on a navigation system: effect of graphical display. In: Proceedings of the driving simulation conference 2010 Europe, Paris, France, pp 199–208

Baumgartner E, Ronellenfitsch A, Reuss H-C, Schramm D (2019) Using a dynamic driving simulator for perception-based powertrain development. Transport Res Part F Traffic Psychol Behav 61:281–290. https://doi.org/10.1016/j.trf.2017.08.012

Bekele MK, Pierdicca R, Frontoni E, Malinverni ES, Gain J (2018) A survey of augmented, virtual, and mixed reality for cultural heritage

Berg LP, Vance JM (2017) Industry use of virtual reality in product design and manufacturing: a survey. Virtual Reality 21:1–17. https://doi.org/10.1007/s10055-016-0293-9

Berthoz A (2000) The brain's sense of movement. Harvard University Press

Bertollini G, Brainer L, Chestnut JA, Oja S, Szczerba J (2010) General motors driving simulator and applications to human machine interface (HMI) development. SAE International, Warrendale, PA

Boer ER (2000) Experiencing the same road twice : a driver centered comparison between simulation and reality. In: Proceedings of the driving simulation conference

Bos JE, MacKinnon SN, Patterson A (2005) Motion sickness symptoms in a ship motion simulator: effects of inside, outside, and no view. Aviat Space Environ Med 76:1111–1118

Boustila S, Capobianco A, Bechmann D (2015) Evaluation of factors affecting distance perception in architectural project review in immersive virtual environments. In: Proceedings of the 21st ACM symposium on virtual reality software and technology, Beijing, China, pp 207–216

Bruder G, Argelaguet F, Olivier A-H, Lécuyer A (2016) CAVE size matters: effects of screen distance and parallax on distance estimation in large immersive display setups. Presence Teleoperators Virtual Environ 25:1–16. https://doi.org/10.1162/PRES_a_00241

Bruschetta M, Cunico D, Chen Y, Beghi A, Minen D (2017) An MPC based multi-sensory cueing algorithm (MSCA) for a high performance driving simulator with active seat. In: Proceedings of the driving simulation conference, pp 65–71

Burns PC, Saluäär D (1999a) Intersections between driving in reality and virtual reality (VR), pp 153–164

Burns PC, Saluäär D (1999b) Intersections between driving in reality and virtual reality (VR). In: DSC'99: driving simulation conference, pp 153–164

Cavallo V (2002) Perceptual distortions when driving in fog. Traffic Transp Stud 2002:965–972. https://doi.org/10.1061/40630(255)135

Cavallo V, Colomb M, Doré J (2001) Distance perception of vehicle rear lights in fog. Hum Factors 43:442–451. https://doi.org/10.1518/001872001775898197

Cavallo V, Dommes A, Vienne F, Dang NT (2016) A street-crossing simulator to study and train pedestrian behaviour. In: Driving simulation conference, Paris, France, pp 195–200

Chapman S (2018) 3D multi-view projection six independent points of view

Chatziastros A, Wallis GM, Bülthoff HH (1999) The effect of field of view and surface texture on driver steering performance

Chen W, Ladeveze N, Clavel C, Mestre D, Bourdot P (2015) User cohabitation in multi-stereoscopic immersive virtual environment for individual navigation tasks. In: 2015 IEEE virtual reality (VR), pp 47–54

Coates N, Ehrette M, Hayes T, Blackham G, Heidet A, Kemeny A (2002) Head-mounted display in driving simulation applications in CARDS. In: Proceedings of the driving simulation conference

Coello Y, Grealy MA (1997) Effect of size and frame of visual field on the accuracy of an aiming movement. Perception 26:287–300. https://doi.org/10.1068/p260287

Colmard O (2018) Connected and autonomous vehicles, a major challenge for the Automotive industry

Colombet F, Dagdelen M, Reymond G, Pere C, Merienne F, Kemeny A (2008) Motion Cueing: what is the impact on the driver's behavior? In: Proceedings of the driving simulation conference Europe. Monaco, pp 171–181

Colombet F, Kemeny A, George P (2016) Motion sickness comparison between a CAVE and a HMD. In: Proceedings of the driving simulation conference, pp 201–208

Combe E, Posselt J, Kemeny A (2008a) 1:1 scale perception in virtual and augmented reality. In: 18th international conference on artificial reality and telexistence, pp 152–160

Combe E, Posselt J, Kemeny A (2008b) Virtual prototype visualization: a size perception study. In: Proceedings of the 5th Nordic conference on Human-computer interaction: building bridges. Association for Computing Machinery, Lund, Sweden, pp 581–582

Cruz-Neira C, Sandin DJ, DeFanti TA, Kenyon RV, Hart JC (1992) The CAVE: audio visual experience automatic virtual environment. Commun ACM 35:64–73

Cutting JE, Vishton PM (1995) Chapter 3—perceiving layout and knowing distances: the integration, relative potency, and contextual use of different information about depth. In: Epstein W, Rogers S (eds) Perception of space and motion. Academic Press, San Diego, pp 69–117

Diels C (2014) Will autonomous vehicles make us sick. Contemporary ergonomics and human factors. Taylor & Francis, pp 301–307

Diels C, Bos JE (2016) Self-driving carsickness. Appl Ergon 53:374–382. https://doi.org/10.1016/j.apergo.2015.09.009

Diels C, Bos JE, Hottelart K, Reilhac P (2016) Motion sickness in automated vehicles: the elephant in the room. In: Road vehicle automation, vol 3. Springer, pp 121–129

Dodgson NA (2005) Autostereoscopic 3D displays. Computer 38:31–36. https://doi.org/10.1109/MC.2005.252

Dogan E, Rahal M-C, Deborne R, Delhomme P, Kemeny A, Perrin J (2017) Transition of control in a partially automated vehicle: effects of anticipation and non-driving-related task involvement. Transp Res Part F Traffic Psychol Behav 46:205–215. https://doi.org/10.1016/j.trf.2017.01.012

Dong X, Stoffregen TA (2010) Postural activity and motion sickness among drivers and passengers in a console video game. Proc Hum Factors Ergon Soc Annual Meet 54:1340–1344. https://doi.org/10.1177/154193121005401808

Drosdol J, Kading W, Panik F (1985) The Daimler-Benz driving simulator. Veh Syst Dyn 14:86–90. https://doi.org/10.1080/00423118508968804

Ellensohn F, Hristakiev D, Schwienbacher M, Venrooij J, Rixen D (2019) Evaluation of an optimization based motion cueing algorithm suitable for online application (accepted). In: Proceedings of the driving simulation conference, driving simulation association

Ernst MO, Bülthoff HH (2004) Merging the senses into a robust percept. Trends Cogn Sci 8:162–169. https://doi.org/10.1016/j.tics.2004.02.002

Fernandes AS, Feiner SK (2016) Combating VR sickness through subtle dynamic field-of-view modification. In: 2016 IEEE symposium on 3D user interfaces (3DUI), pp 201–210

Fröhlich B, Grunst G, Krüger W, Wesche G (1995) The Responsive Workbench: a virtual working environment for physicians. Comput Biol Med 25:301–308. https://doi.org/10.1016/0010-4825(94)00007-D

Fuchs P (2017) Virtual reality headsets—a theoretical and pragmatic approach. CRC Press

Fuchs P, Moreau G, Berthoz A (2003) Le traité de la réalité virtuelle, vol 2. Les Presses de l'École des Mines, Paris

Ghinea M, Frunză D, Chardonnet J-R, Merienne F, Kemeny A (2018) Perception of absolute distances within different visualization systems: HMD and CAVE. In: De Paolis LT, Bourdot P (eds) Augmented reality, virtual reality, and computer graphics. Springer International Publishing, Cham, pp 148–161

Gibson JJ (1950) The perception of the visual world. Houghton Mifflin, Oxford, England

Gibson JJ, Crooks LE (1938) A theoretical field-analysis of automobile-driving. Am J Psychol 51:453–471. https://doi.org/10.2307/1416145

Grabe V, Pretto P, Giordan PR, Bülthoff HH (2010) Influence of display type on drivers' performance in a motion-based driving simulator. In: Proceedings of the driving simulation conference 2010 Europe, pp 81–88

Groen EL, Smaili MH, Hosman RJAW (2007) Perception model analysis of flight simulator motion for a decrab maneuver. J Aircr 44:427–435. https://doi.org/10.2514/1.22872

Hale KS, Stanney KM (2006) Effects of low stereo acuity on performance, presence and sick-ness within a virtual environment. Appl Ergon 37:329–339. https://doi.org/10.1016/j.apergo.2005.06.009

Hallvig D, Anund A, Fors C, Kecklund G, Karlsson JG, Wahde M, Åkerstedt T (2013) Sleepy driving on the real road and in the simulator—a comparison. Accid Anal Prev 50:44–50. https://doi.org/10.1016/j.aap.2012.09.033

Harm DL (2002) Motion sickness neurophysiology, physiological correlates, and treatment. In: Handbook of virtual environments. CRC Press, pp 677–702

Hartfiel B, Stark R (2019) Influence of vestibular cues in head-mounted display-based driving simulators. In: Proceedings of the driving simulation conference 2019 Europe VR, pp 25–32

Hecht J (2016) Optical dreams, virtual reality. Opt Photon News OPN 27:24–31. https://doi.org/10.1364/OPN.27.6.000024

Held RT, Cooper EA, Banks MS (2012) Blur and disparity are complementary cues to depth. Curr Biol 22:426–431. https://doi.org/10.1016/j.cub.2012.01.033

Helland A, Jenssen GD, Lervåg L-E, Westin AA, Moen T, Sakshaug K, Lydersen S, Mørland J, Slørdal L (2013) Comparison of driving simulator performance with real driving after alcohol intake: a randomised, single blind, placebo-controlled, cross-over trial. Accid Anal Prev 53:9–16. https://doi.org/10.1016/j.aap.2012.12.042

Helman S, Reed N (2015) Validation of the driver behaviour questionnaire using behavioural data from an instrumented vehicle and high-fidelity driving simulator. Accid Anal Prev 75:245–251. https://doi.org/10.1016/j.aap.2014.12.008

Hoffman DM, Girshick AR, Akeley K, Banks MS (2008) Vergence–accommodation conflicts hinder visual performance and cause visual fatigue. J Vis 8:33. https://doi.org/10.1167/8.3.33

Howard IP, Rogers BJ (1995) Binocular vision and stereopsis. Oxford University Press, USA

Hua H (2017) Enabling focus cues in head-mounted displays. Proc IEEE 105:805–824. https://doi.org/10.1109/JPROC.2017.2648796

Huang F-C, Chen K, Wetzstein G (2015) The light field stereoscope: immersive computer graphics via factored near-eye light field displays with focus cues. ACM Trans Graph 34:60:1–60:12. https://doi.org/10.1145/2766922

Iskander J, Attia M, Saleh K, Nahavandi D, Abobakr A, Mohamed S, Asadi H, Khosravi A, Lim CP, Hossny M (2019) From car sickness to autonomous car sickness: a review. Transp Res Part F Traffic Psychol Behav 62:716–726

Iskander J, Hossny M, Nahavandi S (2018) A review on ocular biomechanic models for assessing visual fatigue in virtual reality. IEEE Access 6:19345–19361. https://doi.org/10.1109/ACCESS.2018.2815663

Jamson H (2000) Driving simulation validity: issues of field of view and resolution. In: Proceedings of the driving simulation conference, pp 57–64

Jamson H (2001) Image characteristics and their effect on driving simulator validity

Järvenpää T, Salmimaa M (2008) Optical characterization of autostereoscopic 3-D displays. J Soc Inform Display 16:825–833. https://doi.org/10.1889/1.2966444

Käding W, Hoffmeyer F (1995) The advanced Daimler-Benz driving simulator. SAE International, Warrendale, PA

Kalra N, Paddock SM (2016) Driving to safety: how many miles of driving would it take to demonstrate autonomous vehicle reliability? RAND Corporation

Kemeny A (2014) From driving simulation to virtual reality. In: Proceedings of the 2014 virtual reality international conference. Association for Computing Machinery, Laval, France, pp 1–5

Kemeny A (2001) Recent developments in visuo-vestibular restitution of self-motion in driving simulation. In: Proceedings of the driving simulation conference, pp 15–18

Kemeny A (2009) Driving simulation for virtual testing and perception studies. In: Proceedings of the driving simulation conference 2009 Europe, Monaco, pp 15–23

Kemeny A, Colombet F, Denoual T (2015) How to avoid simulation sickness in virtual environments during user displacement. In: The engineering reality of virtual reality 2015. International Society for Optics and Photonics, p 939206

Kemeny A, George P, Mérienne F, Colombet F (2017) New VR navigation techniques to reduce cybersickness. Electron Imaging 2017:48–53

Kemeny A, Panerai F (2003) Evaluating perception in driving simulation experiments. Trends Cogn Sci 7:31–37. https://doi.org/10.1016/S1364-6613(02)00011-6

Kennedy RS, Drexler J, Kennedy RC (2010) Research in visually induced motion sickness. Appl Ergon 41:494–503. https://doi.org/10.1016/j.apergo.2009.11.006

Kennedy RS, Frank LH (1985) A review of motion sickness with special reference to simulator sickness. Canyon Research Group Inc

Kennedy RS, Lane NE, Berbaum KS, Lilienthal MG (1993) Simulator sickness questionnaire: an enhanced method for quantifying simulator sickness. Int J Aviat Psychol 3:203–220. https://doi.org/10.1207/s15327108ijap0303_3

Kennedy RS, Lane NE, Lilienthal MG, Berbaum KS, Hettinger LJ (1992) Profile analysis of simulator sickness symptoms: application to virtual environment systems. Presence Teleoperators Virtual Environ 1:295–301. https://doi.org/10.1162/pres.1992.1.3.295

Kennedy RS, Stanney KM (1996) Postural instability induced by virtual reality exposure: development of a certification protocol. Int J Hum Comput Interact 8:25–47. https://doi.org/10.1080/10447319609526139

Kilteni K, Groten R, Slater M (2012) The sense of embodiment in virtual reality. Presence Teleoperators Virtual Environ 21:373–387. https://doi.org/10.1162/PRES_a_00124

Krueger W, Bohn C-A, Frohlich B, Schuth H, Strauss W, Wesche G (1995) The Responsive Workbench: a virtual work environment. Computer 28:42–48. https://doi.org/10.1109/2.391040

Krueger W, Froehlich B (1994) The Responsive Workbench. IEEE Comput Graph Appl 14:12–15. https://doi.org/10.1109/38.279036

Kruijff E, Swan JE, Feiner S (2010) Perceptual issues in augmented reality revisited. In: 2010 IEEE international symposium on mixed and augmented reality. IEEE, Seoul, Korea (South), pp 3–12

Kuester F, Duchaineau MA, Hamann B, Joy KI, Ma K-L (2000) Designers workbench: toward real-time immersive modeling. In: Stereoscopic Displays and virtual reality systems VII. International Society for Optics and Photonics, pp 464–472

Langlois S (2013) ADAS HMI using peripheral vision. In: Proceedings of the 5th international conference on automotive user interfaces and interactive vehicular applications. Association for Computing Machinery, Eindhoven, Netherlands, pp 74–81

LaViola JJ (2000) A discussion of cybersickness in virtual environments. SIGCHI Bull 32:47–56

Lin JJ-W, Duh HBL, Parker DE, Abi-Rached H, Furness TA (2002) Effects of field of view on presence, enjoyment, memory, and simulator sickness in a virtual environment. Proc IEEE Virtual Reality 2002:164–171

Loomis JM (2001) Looking down is looking up. Nature 414:155–156. https://doi.org/10.1038/35102648

Lyga Y, Lau M, Brandenburg E, Stark R (2020) Validation of immersive design parameters in driving simulation environments. In: Cassenti DN, Scataglini S, Rajulu SL, Wright JL (eds) Advances in simulation and digital human modeling. Springer International Publishing, Cham, pp 136–142

Maria Galeazzi G, Monzani D, Gherpelli C, Covezzi R, Guaraldi GP (2006) Posturographic stabilisation of healthy subjects exposed to full-length mirror image is inversely related to body-image preoccupations. Neurosci Lett 410:71–75. https://doi.org/10.1016/j.neulet.2006.09.077

Mazloumi Gavgani A, Walker FR, Hodgson DM, Nalivaiko E (2018) A comparative study of cybersickness during exposure to virtual reality and "classic" motion sickness: are they different? J Appl Physiol 125:1670–1680. https://doi.org/10.1152/japplphysiol.00338.2018

Merat N, Jamson AH, Lai FCH, Daly M, Carsten OMJ (2014) Transition to manual: driver behaviour when resuming control from a highly automated vehicle. Transp Res Part F Traffic Psychol Behav 27:274–282. https://doi.org/10.1016/j.trf.2014.09.005

Merchant Z, Goetz ET, Cifuentes L, Keeney-Kennicutt W, Davis TJ (2014) Effectiveness of virtual reality-based instruction on students' learning outcomes in K-12 and higher education: a meta-analysis. Comput Educ 70:29–40. https://doi.org/10.1016/j.compedu.2013.07.033

Milgram P, Kishino F (1994) A taxonomy of mixed reality visual displays. IEICE Trans Inf Syst E77-D:1321–1329

Moss JD, Austin J, Salley J, Coats J, Williams K, Muth ER (2011) The effects of display delay on simulator sickness. Displays 32:159–168. https://doi.org/10.1016/j.displa.2011.05.010

Nawrot M (2003) Eye movements provide the extra-retinal signal required for the perception of depth from motion parallax. Vision Res 43:1553–1562. https://doi.org/10.1016/S0042-6989(03)00144-5

Nawrot M, Stroyan K (2012) Integration time for the perception of depth from motion parallax. Vision Res 59:64–71. https://doi.org/10.1016/j.visres.2012.02.007

Nordmark S (1976) Development of a driving simulator. Part report: mathematical vehicle model

Nordmark S, Jansson H, Palmkvist G, Sehammar H (2004) The new VTI driving simulator. Multi purpose moving base with high performance linear motion. In: Proceedings of the driving simulation conference, pp 45–55

Nordmark S, Lidstrom M, Palmkvist G (1984) Moving base driving simulator with wide angle visual system. SAE International, Warrendale, PA

Oliver JH (2018) Virtual and augmented reality: from promise to productivity

Ooi TL, Wu B, He ZJ (2001) Distance determined by the angular declination below the horizon. Nature 414:197–200. https://doi.org/10.1038/35102562

Ostnes R, Abbott V, Lavender S (2004) Visualisation techniques: an overview—part 2. Hydrogr J 114:7

Paes D, Irizarry J (2018) A usability study of an immersive virtual reality platform for building design review: considerations on human factors and user interface. Constr Res Congress 2018:419–428. https://doi.org/10.1061/9780784481264.041

Panerai F, Cornilleau-Pérès V, Droulez J (2002) Contribution of extraretinal signals to the scaling of object distance during self-motion. Percept Psychophys 64:717–731. https://doi.org/10.3758/BF03194739

Panerai F, Droulez J, Kelada J-M, Kemeny A, Balligand E, Favre B (2001) Speed and safety distance control in truck driving: comparison of simulation and real-world environment. In: Proceedings of the driving simulation conference

Perroud B, Gosson R, Colombet F, Regnier S, Collinet J-C, Kemeny A (2020) Contribution of stereoscopy and motion parallax for inter-vehicular distance estimation in driving simulator experiments. In: Proceedings of the driving simulation conference 2020 Europe VR. Driving Simulation Association

Perroud B, Régnier S, Kemeny A, Mérienne F (2019) Model of realism score for immersive VR systems. Transp Res Part F Traffic Psychol Behav 61:238–251. https://doi.org/10.1016/j.trf.2017.08.015

Polcar J, Horejsi P (2013) Knowledge acquisition and cyber sickness: a comparison of VR devices in virtual tours. Science

Prasolova-Førland E, Molka-Danielsen J, Fominykh M, Lamb K (2017) Active learning modules for multi-professional emergency management training in virtual reality. In: 2017 IEEE 6th international conference on teaching, assessment, and learning for engineering (TALE), pp 461–468

Pretto P, Bresciani J-P, Rainer G, Bülthoff HH (2012) Foggy perception slows us down. eLife 1:e00031. https://doi.org/10.7554/eLife.00031

Pretto P, Chatziastros A (2006) Changes in optic flow and scene contrast affect the driving speed. In: Proceedings of the driving simulation conference

Rahimian P, Jiang Y, Yong JP, Franzen L, Plumert JM, Yon JP, Kearney JK (2015) Designing an immersive pedestrian simulator to study the influence of texting and cellphone allerts on road crossing. In: 2015 road safety and simulation international conference

Reason JT, Brand JJ (1975) Motion sickness. Academic Press, Oxford, England

Rebenitsch L, Owen C (2016) Review on cybersickness in applications and visual displays. Virtual Reality 20:101–125. https://doi.org/10.1007/s10055-016-0285-9

Renner RS, Velichkovsky BM, Helmert JR (2013) The perception of egocentric distances in virtual environments—a review. ACM Comput Surv 46:23:1–23:40. https://doi.org/10.1145/2543581.2543590

Reymond G, Kemeny A (2000) Motion cueing in the Renault driving simulator. Veh Syst Dyn 34:249–259. https://doi.org/10.1076/vesd.34.4.249.2059

Reymond G, Kemeny A, Droulez J, Berthoz A (2001) Role of lateral acceleration in curve driving: driver model and experiments on a real vehicle and a driving simulator. Hum Factors 43:483–495. https://doi.org/10.1518/001872001775898188

Riccio GE, Stoffregen TA (1991) An ecological Theory of Motion Sickness and Postural Instability. Ecol Psychol 3:195–240. https://doi.org/10.1207/s15326969eco0303_2

Ritchie ML, Mccoy WK, Welde WL (1968) A study of the relation between forward velocity and lateral acceleration in curves during normal driving. Hum Factors 10:255–258. https://doi.org/10.1177/001872086801000307

Rogers B, Graham M (1979) Motion parallax as an independent cue for depth perception. Perception 8:125–134. https://doi.org/10.1068/p080125

Rolland JP, Holloway RL, Fuchs H (1995) Comparison of optical and video see-through, head-mounted displays. In: Telemanipulator and telepresence technologies. International Society for Optics and Photonics, pp 293–307

Romano R, Markkula G, Giles O, Bean A, Tomlinson A, Sadraei E (2019) Assessment of simulator utility for SCS evaluation. In: Proceedings of the driving simulation conference 2019 Europe VR. Driving Simulation Association, Strasbourg, France, pp 135–142

Ronellenfitsch A, Dong S, Baumgartner E, Reuss H-C, Schramm D (2019) Objective criteria for motion-cueing evaluation. In: Proceedings of the driving simulation conference 2019 Europe VR. Driving Simulation Association, pp 85–91

Rosenblum L, Durbin J, Doyle R, Tate D (1997) The virtual reality Responsive Workbench: applications and experiences. Naval Research Lab, Washington DC

Rushton SK (2004) Egocentric direction and locomotion. In: Vaina LM, Beardsley SA, Rush-ton SK (eds) Optic flow and beyond. Springer, Netherlands, Dordrecht, pp 339–362

Rushton SK, Riddell PM (1999) Developing visual systems and exposure to virtual reality and stereo displays: some concerns and speculations about the demands on accommodation and vergence. Appl Ergon 30:69–78. https://doi.org/10.1016/s0003-6870(98)00044-1

Rushton SK, Salvucci DD (2001) An egocentric account of the visual guidance of locomotion. Trends Cogn Sci 5:6–7. https://doi.org/10.1016/S1364-6613(00)01562-X

Ruthenbeck GS, Reynolds KJ (2015) Virtual reality for medical training: the state-of-the-art. J Simul 9:16–26. https://doi.org/10.1057/jos.2014.14

Sadraei E, Romano R, Merat N, Garcia de Pedro J, Lee YM, Madigan R, Uzondu C, Lyu W, Tomlinson A (2020) Vehicle-pedestrian interaction: a distributed simulation study. In: Proceedings of the driving simulation conference. Antibes, France

Sawabe T, Kanbara M, Hagita N (2016) Diminished reality for acceleration—motion sickness reduction with vection for autonomous driving. In: 2016 IEEE international symposium on mixed and augmented reality (ISMAR-Adjunct). IEEE, pp 297–299

Schmieder H, Nagel K, Schoener H-P (2017) Enhancing a driving simulator with a 3D-stereo projection system. In: Proceedings of the driving simulator conference

Sheridan TB (1992) Musings on telepresence and virtual presence. Presence Teleoperators Virtual Environ 1:120–126. https://doi.org/10.1162/pres.1992.1.1.120

Sherman WR, Craig AB (2003) Understanding virtual reality: interface, application, and design. Morgan Kaufmann Publishers, Amsterdam, Boston

Sivak M (1996) The information that drivers use: is it indeed 90% visual? Perception 25:1081–1089. https://doi.org/10.1068/p251081

Sivak M, Schoettle B (2015) Motion sickness in self-driving vehicles. University of Michigan, Ann Arbor, Transportation Research Institute

Slater M (2009) Place illusion and plausibility can lead to realistic behaviour in immersive virtual environments. Philos Trans R Soc B Biol Sci 364:3549–3557. https://doi.org/10.1098/rstb.2009.0138

Slater M, Wilbur S (1997) A framework for immersive virtual environments (FIVE): speculations on the role of presence in virtual environments. Presence Teleoperators Virtual Environ 6:603–616. https://doi.org/10.1162/pres.1997.6.6.603

Snowden RJ, Stimpson N, Ruddle RA (1998) Speed perception fogs up as visibility drops. Nature 392:450–450. https://doi.org/10.1038/33049

Sovani S (2017) Simulation accelerates development of autonomous driving. ATZ Worldw 119:24–29. https://doi.org/10.1007/s38311-017-0088-y

Stoffregen TA, Smart LJ (1998) Postural instability precedes motion sickness. Brain Res Bull 47:437–448. https://doi.org/10.1016/S0361-9230(98)00102-6

Strobl M, Huesmann A (2004) High flexibility : an important issue for user studies in driving simulation. In: Proceedings of the driving simulation conference, pp 57–65

Sutherland IE (1968) A head-mounted three dimensional display. In: Proceedings of the December 9–11, 1968, fall joint computer conference, part I. Association for Computing Machinery, San Francisco, California, pp 757–764

Thompson WB, Willemsen P, Gooch AA, Creem-Regehr SH, Loomis JM, Beall AC (2004) Does the quality of the computer graphics matter when judging distances in visually immersive environments? Presence Teleoperators Virtual Environ 13:560–571. https://doi.org/10.1162/105474 6042545292

Treisman M (1977) Motion sickness: an evolutionary hypothesis. Science 197:493–495. https://doi.org/10.1126/science.301659

Uliano KC, Kennedy RS, Lambert EY (1986) Asynchronous visual delays and the development of simulator sickness. Proc Hum Factors Soc Annu Meet 30:422–426. https://doi.org/10.1177/154 193128603000502

Vaillant J, Vuillerme N, Janvy A, Louis F, Juvin R, Nougier V (2004) Mirror versus stationary cross feedback in controlling the center of foot pressure displacement in quiet standing in elderly subjects. Arch Phys Med Rehabil 85:1962–1965. https://doi.org/10.1016/j.apmr.2004.02.019

van Leeuwen TD, Cleij D, Pool DM, Mulder M, Bülthoff HH (2019) Time-varying perceived motion mismatch due to motion scaling in curve driving simulation. Transp Res Part F Traffic Psychol Behav 61:84–92. https://doi.org/10.1016/j.trf.2018.05.022

Venrooij J, Pretto P, Katliar M, Nooij S, Nesti A, Lächele M, de Winkel K, Cleij D, Bülthoff HH (2015) Perception-based motion cueing: validation in driving simulation. In: Proceedings of the driving simulation conference Europe, Tuebingen, Germany, pp 153–162

Vovk A, Wild F, Guest W, Kuula T (2018) Simulator sickness in augmented reality training using the Microsoft HoloLens. In: Proceedings of the 2018 CHI conference on human factors in computing systems, pp 1–9

Watt SJ, Akeley K, Ernst MO, Banks MS (2005) Focus cues affect perceived depth. J Vis 5:834–862. https://doi.org/10.1167/5.10.7

Weech S, Kenny S, Barnett-Cowan M (2019) Presence and cybersickness in virtual reality are negatively related: a review. Front Psychol 10. https://doi.org/10.3389/fpsyg.2019.00158

Weyrich M, Drews P (1999) An interactive environment for virtual manufacturing: the virtual workbench. Comput Ind 38:5–15. https://doi.org/10.1016/S0166-3615(98)00104-3

Wienrich C, Weidner CK, Schatto C, Obremski D, Israel JH (2018) A virtual nose as a rest-frame—the impact on simulator sickness and game experience. In: 2018 10th international conference on virtual worlds and games for serious applications (VS-Games), pp 1–8

Wierwille WW, Casali JG, Repa BS (1983) Driver steering reaction time to abrupt-onset crosswinds, as measured in a moving-base driving simulator. Hum Factors 25:103–116. https://doi.org/10.1177/001872088302500110

Wintersberger P, Frison A-K, Riener A, Sawitzky T von (2019) Fostering user acceptance and trust in fully automated vehicles: evaluating the potential of augmented reality. Presence Virtual Augment Reality 27:46–62. https://doi.org/10.1162/pres_a_00320

Yan JK (1985) Advances in computer-generated imagery for flight simulation. IEEE Comput Graph Appl 5:37–51. https://doi.org/10.1109/MCG.1985.276213

Yao R, Heath T, Davies A, Forsyth T, Mitchell N, Hoberman P (2014) Oculus VR best practices guide. Oculus VR 4

Zeeb E (2010) Daimler's new full-scale, high-dynamic driving simulator–a technical overview. Actes INRETS 157–165

Zhang B, Wilschut ES, Willemsen DMC, Martens MH (2019) Transitions to manual control from highly automated driving in non-critical truck platooning scenarios. Transp Res Part F Traffic Psychol Behav 64:84–97. https://doi.org/10.1016/j.trf.2019.04.006

# Chapter 2
# Self-motion Perception and Cybersickness

**Abstract** Understanding self-motion perception is essential to design and apply countermeasures against cybersickness. This section provides introductory knowledge of motion perception, carried out by our visual systems and vestibular as well as kinesthetic organs. Vection and optic flow give elementary sensations of motion, but a partial or incorrect integration of all the necessary sensorial information gives rise to motion sickness. The main theories explaining motion sickness and the various factors affecting its effects are shortly presented with the most essential information on the underlying mechanisms and the necessary details on their links with motion perception in virtual worlds and the potential motion and VR induced sickness effects. Since motion sickness is one of the most observed origins of cybersickness when moving in the virtual world using virtual navigation tools, this section gives essential information on its effects as well as the age, gender, or social parameters that influence it. Finally, the technological parameters, affecting motion and VR induced sickness effects, are shortly introduced, allowing for a comprehensive understanding of the visual and motion rendering systems. The latter are described in the following chapter.

## 2.1 Sensory Organs

### 2.1.1 Visual System

Vision is the predominant sense in human beings: a crucial part of the human cerebral cortex is devoted to the analysis of the visual world (Berthoz 2000; Bear et al. 2016). Thanks to the mastery of this sense, humans have been able to develop mental mechanisms to predict the trajectory of objects and the course of events in space and time and to create new means of communication and the world of art, among other things. At present, humans are even able to recreate virtual but realistic and confounding environments and create the illusion of being in these worlds mainly through visual displays and virtual reality technologies. The eye is a remarkable organ capable of detecting things ranging from the size of an insect to that of a galaxy at the

A. Kemeny et al., *Getting Rid of Cybersickness*,
https://doi.org/10.1007/978-3-030-59342-1_2

other end of the universe. This section aims to describe in more detail of how the eye works, especially in spatial perception (speed and distance perception), observation, and orientation—these aspects of visual perception being the most used in Virtual Reality (VR) and simulation.

### 2.1.1.1  General Description of the Eye

In the center of the eye's visible part is the pupil (see Fig. 2.1), an opening that allows light to penetrate inside of the eye. The iris—a circular muscle whose pigmentation gives the eye its color—has the role of controlling the opening of the pupil. The pupil and iris are covered by a liquid: the aqueous humor, contained by the cornea. The eye's first interface with the outside world—the cornea—does not contain any blood vessels so as not to have any influence on the image of the outside world. Furthermore, to preserve the sharpness of its surface, it is covered with a thin layer of tears spread evenly by the eyelids. Finally, the cornea is in continuity with the sclera, commonly called the white of the eye, on which the three ocular muscles that allow the eye to rotate in its orbit are fixed.

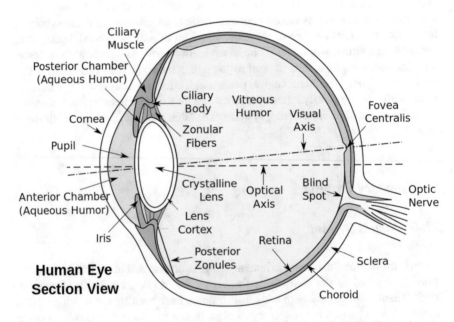

**Fig. 2.1** Human eye, section view. https://commons.wikimedia.org/wiki/File:Eyesection.svg. Based on Eyesection.gif, by en:User_talk:Sathiyam2k. Vectorization and some modifications by user:ZStardust/Public domain

**Fig. 2.2** Vergence angle of
the eyes depends on the
distance to the observed
object and provides a depth
cue

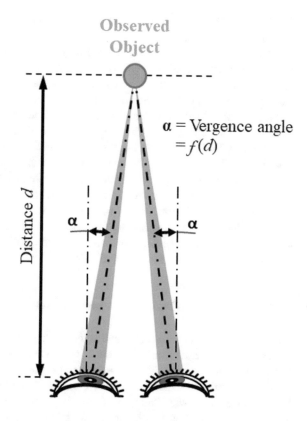

Observed
Object

$\alpha$ = Vergence angle
= $f(d)$

Distance $d$

$\alpha$

$\alpha$

### 2.1.1.2 Eye Orientation and Vergence Mechanism

The orientation of the three ocular muscles is close to that of the semicircular canals
of the vestibular system (see next Sect. 2.1.2). As we will see in the visuo-vestibular
coupling section, this is an evolutionary result common to all vertebrates to ease the
mechanism of eye stabilization (vestibulo-ocular reflex). These muscles also allow
the eye to rotate and follow a specific target. Depending on the distance to this target,
the eyes will have to rotate inward toward the nose (converge) or outward toward
the ears (diverge). This vergence movement and orientation of the eyes give a depth
cue on the distance to the observed object (see Fig. 2.2) (Grant 1942; Von Hofsten
1976).

### 2.1.1.3 Accommodation

When light, after passing through the pupil, enters the eye, it reaches the inner surface
of the eye—the retina. It is in the deepest layer of the retina that the photoreceptors
are found that will transform light intensity into nerve impulses (Remington 2012).

These impulses are sent to the brain via the optic nerve, which exits at the back of the eye.

The lens of the eye (crystalline lens) plays the same role as a camera lens in a camera—namely, it provides a sharp image regardless of the distance of the object at which the eye is looking. The eye lens is a transparent surface located behind the iris and is suspended between ligaments attached to the ciliary muscles. The contraction or relaxation of these muscles will stretch or bulge the lens, resulting in a change in its convergence. This way, the image of the outside world will be clear on the retina. This mechanism is called accommodation and, in addition to having a clear image, it makes it possible to obtain information on the distance at which the object being viewed is located (Fisher and Ciuffreda 1988). In VR environments, this distance information from accommodation can sometimes be in contradiction with the distance information from eye vergence, as illustrated in Fig. 1.3, due to the accommodation being done on the display screen instead of the virtual object itself. This is called the vergence-accommodation conflict and is one of the supposed causes of cybersickness (Shibata et al. 2011).

### 2.1.1.4  Central and Peripheral Vision in the Retina

The retina has the same role in the eye as the photographic film in a camera. However, central and peripheral retinas do not have the same physiological characteristics and composition, thus giving different roles and purposes to these different parts of the eyes. Proper understanding of their diverse features allows for better designing of VR interfaces (e.g., where and how to display each type of information) and visual display setups (e.g., how much horizontal Field Of View (FOV) needs to be covered, depending on the task).

An ophthalmoscopic examination of the eye reveals the macula—an area in the center of the retina. No large blood vessels of any size pass through this area, thus making the central vision of the eye of better "quality" than peripheral vision (Remington 2012). The fovea—a 2 mm-diameter spot with a thinner retina—is in the center of this macula (see Fig. 2.1). Geometrically, it is also the area diametrically opposite the pupil, in which the images corresponding to the central vision are formed. Fovea has a diameter of 5.2°, whereas the macula's diameter is around 17° (Strasburger et al. 2011). The complete human visual field covers approximately 200°–220° horizontally with 120° covered by both eyes, and 130°–135° vertically. Figure 2.3 illustrates these different fields of view.

The photoreceptors can be distinguished between cones and rods, which are unequally distributed over the retina. The central retina has a high concentration of cones and a virtual absence of rods, making it the preferred area for color detection and high-light vision (day vision). On the other hand, the peripheral retina has a large number of rods and is almost devoid of cones. It is therefore mainly used for low-light vision (night vision).

The retina has a laminar organization in three main layers. At the deepest side of the retina (i.e., the farthest from the vitreous humor) is the outer nuclear layer, in which the

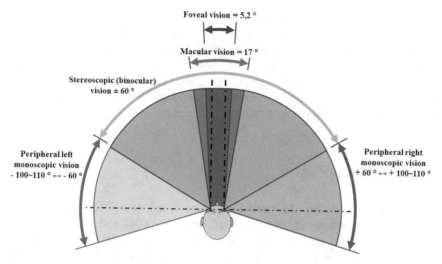

**Fig. 2.3** Illustration of the horizontal fields of view: foveal vision, macular vision, stereoscopic (binocular) vision, and peripheral monoscopic vision (left and right)

photoreceptors are located. The cells contained in the two other layers are not directly sensitive to light and have a role of transmission of the nerve impulses emitted by the photoreceptors. On each retina layer, the number of cells decreases, thus making some signal processing before being transmitted to the brain. The ganglion cells on the upper layer of the retina are the only ones that transmit information to the brain, based on the principle of action potentials,[1] through the optic nerve formed with their axons.

Ganglion cells can be classified into several large families. In studies conducted on cat retinas (Enroth-Cugell and Robson 1984), cells are classified into α, β, γ, or δ according to their size or into W, X, and Y according to their visual response characteristic. This classification inspired the work initiated by Watanabe and Rodieck (1989) and later continued by Kaplan and Bernadete (2001) on macaque retinas, closer to human retinas. These studies highlighted the existence of two main types of ganglion cells: large M-type cells (from *magnus*, "large" in Latin) and smaller P-type cells (for *parvus*, "small" in Latin). Approximately, 90% of ganglion cells are P-type and 5% M-type, the remaining 5% being yet uncharacterized ganglion cells.

Beyond size, they also differ in their distribution (Curcio and Allen 1990). M-type cells are mainly present in the peripheral retina. P-type cells—the majority type—are present throughout the retina, but there is some concentration around the fovea.

P-type and M-type lymph node cells also differ in response (Kaplan and Bernadete 2001). M cells propagate their action potentials at a higher rate than P cells. In

---

[1]At rest, the ganglion cells emit action potentials at a base frequency through their axons. This is called the tonic discharge. When they are excited, the frequency of emission of their action potentials increases. On the contrary, when they are inhibited, the frequency of emission of their action potentials decreases.

addition, they respond to a stimulus with a brief burst of action potentials, regardless of the duration of the stimulus. Conversely, P cells respond as long as the stimulus works. M cells thus seem predisposed to motion detection, while P cells are more sensitive to the details and shape of the stimulus. When adding the distribution and properties of the photoreceptors and the ganglion cells over the retina, the central vision is used for shape and color detection, while peripheral vision is used for motion detection and night vision.

### 2.1.2  Vestibular System

Located in the inner ear, the vestibular system is an organ used to perceive the position and movements of the head (Graf and Klam 2006), and its functioning is mainly based on hair cells. It is composed of two types of organs: three semicircular canals and two otolithic organs, the utricle and the saccule (see Fig. 2.4). We will see that these two types of organs have similarities in their functioning and serve to provide the brain with spatial information about the position and movements of the

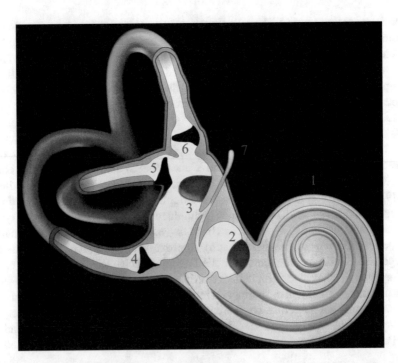

**Fig. 2.4**  Human inner ear description. 1. Cochlea. 2. Saccule. 3. Utricle. 4. Posterior ductus ampulla. 5. External ductus ampulla. 6. Superior ductus ampulla. 7. ductus endolymphaticus. https://commons.wikimedia.org/wiki/File:Oreille_Interne.png. Didier Descouens/CC BY-SA (https://creativecommons.org/licenses/by-sa/3.0)

head. However, the types of information perceived are quite distinct: the semicircular canals react to the angular accelerations of the head, while the otolithic organs react to linear accelerations as well as to the inclination of the head.

The vestibular system, by providing information on the position and orientation of the head, gives a sense of balance and is used to coordinate the head and eye movements, as well as to adjust the body's posture. The vestibular system intervenes permanently and unconsciously (through several reflexes) to control the balance. We only become aware of its existence in the event of a strong or prolonged conflict with the other senses, such as motion sickness, alcohol poisoning, and dizziness. It should also be noted that vestibular cues cannot be interrupted as can visual cues be by closing the eyes, for example, or sound cues by closing the ears.

### 2.1.2.1 Semicircular Canals

The semicircular canals are sensitive to the rotational movements of the head. There are three of them per vestibular system (horizontal canal, anterior canal, and posterior canal) because, as we evolve in a three-dimensional universe, it is essential to be able to perceive all the rotations of the head.

The semicircular canals are contained in orthogonal planes two by two. Contrary to what one might think at first glance, these planes are not parallel to the main body planes (horizontal, frontal, and sagittal). The horizontal channel is inclined at an angle of 25°–30°, and the anterior and posterior channels are inclined at an angle of about 45°. There is no explanation yet as to the reason for these inclinations. However, the ocular muscles are oriented in the same way; changing the reference mark for eye movement during the vestibulo-ocular reflex is thus easier and can be done more quickly (Graf and Klam 2006).

The semicircular canals, which are made of small pipes of about 6 mm in diameter, are filled with a viscous liquid, the endolymph. At the base of these channels is a protrusion—the ampulla crest—in which the hair cells are located. In the event of rotation, the endolymph tends by inertia to remain motionless in the terrestrial landmark and thus moves in the opposite direction of the rotation of the channel in a landmark linked to the canal. When the endolymph moves, it exerts a pressure force on the eyelashes, which are then tilted. Depending on this inclination, the nerve message delivered by the hair cells to the brain via the vestibular nerve is then modified. Like the ganglion cells of the retina, hair cells send information to the brain in the form of action potentials. Information about eyelash tilt is therefore transmitted to the brain by a frequency-modulated signal.

Although semicircular canals are indeed sensitive to angular accelerations, they are sometimes considered in the literature as sensors providing angular velocity information. In the response models provided by van Egmond et al. (1949) and Heerspink et al. (2005), semicircular channels achieve both integration and low-pass filtering. Thus, the perceived angular velocity corresponds to a low-pass filtering of the angular velocity of the head. We thus have a first explanation as to why semicircular channels are considered as angular velocity sensors rather than angular acceleration sensors. In this case, they only perform a low-pass filtering of the angular velocity of the head.

Response analysis of the semicircular canals also reveals the significant inertia (in the order of 20 s) of the semicircular channels when the angular acceleration is canceled, i.e., when the angular velocity is constant. Since the head is rarely stationary (or at a constant angular velocity) for such a long time, it is rare for the semicircular canals not to return any information. This feature has also reinforced the idea that semicircular canals can be considered as angular velocity sensors.

### 2.1.2.2  Otolithic Organs

The utricle and saccule are the two otolithic organs of the vestibular system that make the perception of rectilinear accelerations and the inclination of the head possible. Like semicircular canals, otolithic organs have hair cells that function by the emission of action potentials. Each otolithic organ has a sensory area called the macula (not to be confused with the macula of the eye). The utricle is generally horizontal, while the saccule is more or less vertically oriented. In each of these maculae, the orientation of the hair cells is not identical in each place such that each movement of the head will excite some hair cells, inhibit others, and have no effect on the rest. In addition, this phenomenon will be found symmetrically in the saccule (or utricle) of the other ear.

The maculae of the utricle and saccule work in the same way and are composed of three layers. The lower layer is formed by the bases of hair cells and support cells; it is interdependent with the vestibular system, and thus also with the head during its movements. The upper layer is composed of small calcium carbonate crystals called "otoliths" (from a Greek word meaning "ear stone"), from 1 to 5 μm in diameter. Otoliths have a higher density than the endolymph surrounding them. Finally, the intermediate layer linking the other two layers is made of a gelatinous cap in which the eyelashes of the hair cells are embedded.

When the head is accelerated, otoliths tend by inertia to remain still in the terrestrial reference frame and move in the opposite direction of the head movement in a reference frame related to the vestibular system. The upper and lower layers exert a shear force on the intermediate layer, which has the effect of tilting the eyelashes. Similarly, when the head is tilted, the otoliths move down by gravity, and the upper and lower layers, again, exert a shearing force on the intermediate layer, causing the eyelashes to tilt. The otolithic organs are thus indistinctly excited by an acceleration in the horizontal plane or an inclination of the head.

Unlike semicircular canals, which, as we have seen previously, have a rather long response time, otolithic organs have a much shorter response time. The transfer function of the otoliths was modeled by Wentink et al. (2006) as the sum of the undergone acceleration and its high-pass filtering. This high-pass part of the response represents human sensitivity to the jerk—namely, the time derivative of acceleration. In most cases, the jerk acts as a kind of alert index (Berthoz 2000) and is usually clearly perceived by humans. The larger the jerk—namely, the faster the acceleration changes—the more intense the response of the otolithic organs will be.

### 2.1.2.3   Detection Thresholds

The functioning of otolithic organs and semicircular canals is not perfect: there is a detection threshold below which they are not activated. For linear accelerations, the threshold is around 0.05 m/s². For longitudinal movements, it would be 0.03 m/s², according to Hamann et al. (2001), 0.048 m/s², according to Gianna et al. (1996), and 0.063 m/s², according to Benson et al. (1986). Benson et al. (1986) have also measured a threshold of 0.057 m/s² for lateral displacements and a threshold of 0.154 m/s² for vertical displacements.

For angular accelerations, Clark and Stewart (1968) place this threshold around 0.11°/s², while Bringoux et al. (2002) place it between 0.2 and 2°/s². Benson et al. (1989) measured this threshold as a function of the axis of rotation and raised a threshold of 1.4°/s² for rotations around the vertical axis (yaw rotation), 2.04°/s² about the anteroposterior axis (roll rotation) and, finally, 2.07°/s² around the lateral axis (pitch rotation). By jointly presenting a visual motion, Groen and Bles (2004) obtained a higher detection threshold of 3°/s for pitch rotations.

In a simulator based on a robotic arm (see Fig. 3.7), Nesti et al. (2012) showed that within a dynamic driving scenario and with pure tilt motion, the roll-rate threshold can be raised to a much higher value (about 5.2°/s) and suggested a high tilt rate threshold of 6°/s in driving simulation. For roll-tilt rendering in an active driving scenario, recent values seem to confirm this threshold (6°/s for Pretto et al. (2014), and 5°/s for Fang et al. (2014)). For pitch tilt rendering, Colombet et al. (2015) found an acceptability rate threshold of 6°/s, as well as a strong influence of rotational acceleration on the driver's acceptability if the used rotational rate is greater than 5°/s. Although most studies focus on rotational rate, it seems that for the same rotational speed, having a higher rotational acceleration to reach this speed decreases the detection threshold.

Moreover, these thresholds are apparently not constant: they seem to vary not only according to individuals, understandably, but also according to the duration of the stimulus. Rodenburg et al. (1981), for example, found that the threshold of angular acceleration perception in the dark could be

$a_{threshold} = \frac{0.22}{1-e^{-\frac{t_s}{14.5}}} °/s^2$, where $t_s$ is the duration of the stimulus.

### 2.1.2.4   Conclusion

The vestibular system acts as an inertial unit, providing information on acceleration, inclination, and rotation of the head. As with the retina with visual information, we see that initial processing of gravito-inertial information is performed before it is sent back to the brain. Thus, the information returned by the semicircular canals does not correspond to the angular acceleration, but rather to a high-pass filtering of the head's rotational speed. Specifically, they return information close to the rotation speed when it varies, and no information when it remains constant (whether it is null or not).

Concerning the otolithic organs, it appears that the returned signal corresponds to the linear accelerations of the head to which a high-pass filtering of these same accelerations is added. The signal is then magnified following a sudden change in acceleration—namely, when the jerk is large. One possible interpretation of this phenomenon is that the otolithic organs act as a kind of alarm activated in the event of a major jerk to trigger reflex mechanisms—for example, during a fall.

## 2.2  Proprioception and Visuo-vestibular Coupling

Proprioception is the sense of self-movement, including body position and balance, which is sometimes considered as a 6th sense (Tuthill and Azim 2018), though many consider vestibular perception as the 6th sense (Berthoz 2000). Many also distinguish proprioception (perception of body position) from kinesthesia (perception of the body's movement through space), which interacts with the information provided by the vestibular system (Sousa et al. 2012). The somatosensory system, which includes not only proprioception but also the sense of touch, strongly interacts with all the motion perception modalities (Hagner and Webster 1988).

Proprioception and accompanying neuromuscular feedback mechanisms provide crucial information for the establishment and maintenance of body stability or, for example, to localize one's hand—namely, to find out its position relative to the body (van Beers et al. 1999; Bove et al. 2009). Indeed, the displacement of images on the retina may be induced by the movement of the observer or by the environment, and the subject's proprioceptive functions can only explain why he or she is able to maintain stability when moving (Berthoz 1974). Specifically, the Central Nervous System (CNS) integrates the proprioception with all the other sensory systems, especially vision and the vestibular system, to create an overall representation of body position, movement, and kinetics. The properties and applied mechanisms are still a subject of intense research. Proprioception thus plays a crucial role in VR too and completes the role of visual and vestibular cues necessary to ensure body stability. Hence, its role is crucial to understand the underlying mechanism of cybersickness.

### 2.2.1  Optic Flow

Optic flow, defined as the visual motion experienced while walking, driving, or flying, has been extensively investigated (Lappe et al. 1999; Li and Warren 2002) and is thought to play a dominant role in the control of heading (Lappe et al. 1999) and collision detection (Lee 1980; Lappe et al. 1999; Gray and Regan 2000). Nevertheless, if the very structure of the flow was put forward by Warren et al. (Warren et al. 1988; Warren and Hannon 1988) for the control of the direction of movement in natural environments, recent studies (Wann and Land 2000; Bruggeman et al. 2007) indicate that egocentric heading may also play an important role. The optic-flow strategy, in which one aligns the direction of locomotion or "heading" specified by optic flow with the visual goal, mostly works in visually rich environments, while the egocentric-direction strategy, in which one aligns the locomotor axis with the perceived egocentric direction of the goal, is more suitable in sparse environments (Bruggeman et al. 2007).

Optic flow itself does not give information about the absolute distance to an object and locomotion speed. Rather, it can be used for time measurements, also called time-to-contact (Tresilian 1995; Lee et al. 2009), namely, the time before reaching a specific object if no action on the trajectory or the speed is performed. However, under certain conditions, optic flow proved to be a reliable cue to estimate travel distances (Bremmer and Lappe 1999; Redlick et al. 2001).

Furthermore, we tend to fixate points of the forthcoming trajectory during natural locomotion. When driving a vehicle, we use the angle between the tangent point of the inner lane markings and the car's heading direction, as it was first suggested in a now well-known paper (Land and Lee 1994). As it is proportional to the required steering angle, it is thus an easy strategy to use by the driver, as studied in driving simulators in various conditions (Boer 1996; Reymond et al. 2001; Coutton-Jean et al. 2009) or to be used in autonomous vehicles control laws (Taylor et al. 1999).

## 2.2.2 Vection

### 2.2.2.1 Definition of Vection

Vection is a powerful phenomenon of induction of self-motion by visual stimulation and is central in all VR and driving simulation experiences. The train illusion is the best known and most representative example of this phenomenon. When finding ourselves in a train stopped at the platform and when the neighboring train starts, we have the impression that it is our train that is moving (see Fig. 2.5). Vection is often considered a perceptive illusion because a clean movement is perceived while the subject is objectively motionless. Vection would then be an error of perception committed by the brain. However, many authors consider it a natural perception process of the brain.

It is thus understandable that vection may be considered as central in VR and driving simulation. While displaying an image computed from a moving point of view in a virtual world, vection will induce the viewers to believe that they are moving in the virtual world while being objectively not moving in the same manner. This discrepancy between the visually perceived motion induced by vection and the motion being physically sensed by the vestibular system is the main sensorial

**Fig. 2.5** The train illusion,
illustrating the vection
phenomenon

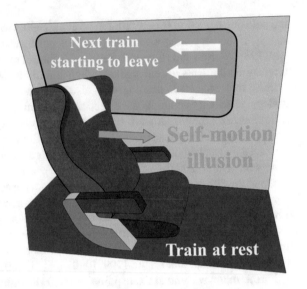

conflict (but not the only one) generally referred to as visuo-vestibular conflict and
can lead to cybersickness (Reason and Brand 1975). It is then crucial to understand
the underlying mechanisms of vection to prevent undesired effects.

Gibson was the first to question the illusory side of vection. In his ecological
approach to visual perception (Gibson 1979), he explains that an observer who uses
their retina to measure a movement of the environment relative to themselves necessarily perceives themselves in movement because in ecological (i.e., natural) conditions, the environment is always stationary. The illusion produced on a flight or
driving simulator is thus never an illusion in an ecological situation.

Furthermore, according to Dichgans and Brandt (1978), the vestibular nuclei are
also activated during vection, following the same temporal evolution as the sensation
of proper motion. As the signal returned by the vestibular system is extinguished at
a given speed (see Chap. 2, Sect. 2.1.2), this finding on the activation of vestibular
nuclei has led to the hypothesis that vection plays a complementary role to vestibular
information. Specifically, vection does not appear instantaneously, and its latency is
consistent with the hypothesis of complementarity between vision and the vestibular
system.

### 2.2.2.2  Establishment of Vection

Vection is not an instantaneous phenomenon: it appears with a latency varying from
1 to 10 s. It becomes exclusive after 5 to 15 s; we then speak of saturated vection.
Dichgans and Brandt (1978) report that vection can last up to 30 s after the stimulus
disappears by extinguishing the light. These values were obtained in circular vection
(rotational movement) using textured cylinders rotating around the subject. Berhoz

et al. (1975) found similar results in linear vection (translational motion). It has been found that when vestibular stimulation is consistent with visual movement, the vection's lag, as well as the saturated vection establishment time, are reduced. These results were obtained both in circular vection (Groen et al. 1999) and in linear vection (Berthoz et al. 1975). They thus reveal the importance of physical restitution in both driving simulation and VR.

The smaller the vection's lag, the smaller the period during which the simulation is not perceived as realistic. On the other hand, when vestibular stimulation is in conflict with the visual movement, the circular vection seems little or not at all affected (Groen et al. 1999), while the detection and identification of the direction of movement appear to be strongly degraded in linear vection (Berthoz et al. 1975). A study by Pavard and Berthoz (1977) demonstrates that the presentation of vestibular stimulation can lead to the illusion of the visual flow slowing down or even stopping.

The sensation of self-motion movement is thus the result of the interaction between visual and inertial stimulus. In addition, it has optimal characteristics when these two stimuli are coherent. Conflict results in either degradation of the vection or a choice of a dominant modality. Furthermore, conflicts between visual and vestibular information can also cause the occurrence of motion sickness (Hettinger et al. 1990) or cybersickness (see Sect. 2.3).

Cognitive factors may also influence the establishment of vection, as recently demonstrated (Palmisano and Chan 2004; Wright et al. 2006). The results of these studies indicate that a priori knowledge of the possibility of physical movement consistent with visual movement improves the credibility of the movement but has no effect on the latency of the vection. Similarly, Riecke et al. (2006) demonstrate that the use of a photo-realistic environment helps to reduce the latency of the vection.

### 2.2.2.3 Influences of Central and Peripheral Vision

Numerous studies have been conducted on the influences of central and peripheral vision on vection and its potentially strong impact on the visual display setup to use and the user's field of view that we want to cover to favor or limit the apparition of vection. Several hypotheses emanate from these studies that Bardy et al. (1999) suggest classifying in three categories: peripheral dominance, differential sensitivity to radial flow, and retinal invariance.

The peripheral dominance hypothesis by Dichgans and Brandt (1978) postulates that the stimuli in peripheral vision would be preponderant in the perception of self-motion, as opposed to the central visual information mainly involved in the perception of object movement. This hypothesis is the most widespread today and is also based on the anatomical study of the eye (see Chap. 2, Sect. 2.1.1).

The differential sensitivity hypothesis, defended by Warren and Kurtz (1992), postulates that the influence of central and peripheral vision on self-motion perception depends in fact on their functional sensitivity; namely, the peripheral retina would be rather sensitive to lamellar flow, whereas central vision would be preferentially sensitive to radial flow.

Finally, the retinal invariance hypothesis goes against the first two by postulating that central and peripheral vision have an equivalent role in the perception of movement. For example, Crowell and Banks (1993), by using radial and lamellar flows presented at different eccentricities, demonstrate that central and peripheral vision have the same sensitivity to the perception of movement. Post (1988) shows that, for circular vection, eccentricity has no influence on it as long as the surface of the stimulus remains constant. Tarita-Nistor et al. (2006) find similar results for linear vection, but only if a fixation point is added to the stimulus. According to the authors, in the absence of this fixation point, peripheral vision has more effect than central vision for inducing vection.

In view of these different hypotheses on the respective influences of central and peripheral vision on vection, it seems difficult to find a definite conclusion. Moreover, the lack of consensus both at the level of the very definition of the fields of vision in terms of amplitude and the experimental paradigms used does not allow for an easy comparison of the different experimental results. However, we can retain that stimulation of the central vision under certain conditions can generate the phenomenon of vection and that the stimulation of peripheral vision would seem to favor the emergence of the sensation of proper movement.

### 2.2.3    Vestibulo-ocular Reflex

#### 2.2.3.1    Impact of Vestibulo-ocular Reflex in Virtual Reality

In real as well as the virtual world, to keep a clear vision while walking or, more generally, during any locomotion, or simply to look at an object from different viewing angles, the vision needs to be stabilized. The stabilization process aims at keeping the image of the world on the retina long enough so that the visual system can process it and thus correctly perceive the surrounding world. As seen before, the central vision (macula of the retina) is used for shape and color detection, whereas peripheral vision is used for motion detection and night vision (Kaplan and Bernadete 2001). The stabilization process of the eye is thus also used to keep the observed object in the central vision. This process is handled by the Vestibulo-Ocular Reflexes (VORs)—a set of eye movements countering head and whole-body motion by rotating the eye in the opposite direction (Angelaki 2009). The vestibular system triggers them, so they also work for external motion stimulation and do not depend on visual input.

In most Virtual Reality environments, the user's head position is tracked to compute the image to display for the correct point of view and orientation. The overall latency between the user's actual motion and the resulting update on the visual display is called the Motion To Photon (MTP) latency (Zhao et al. 2017). If the MTP latency of the used setup is higher than the eye's stabilization process latency, it may result in an unstable world perception followed by cybersickness. Specifically, if the MTP latency is too high, the VORs will compensate the head's motion before the image on the visual display, and the virtual world (in VR) or the

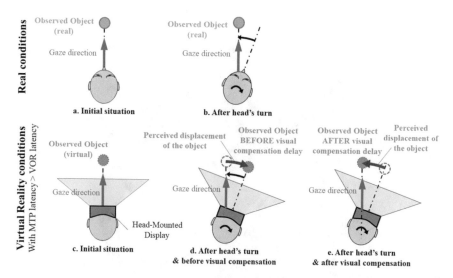

**Fig. 2.6** Impact of display latency on gaze stabilization by VOR. In the initial situations (**a** and **c**), the gaze is directed toward the observed object (real or virtual). When the head turns (**b** and **d**), the eyes rotate in the opposite direction to keep the gaze toward the observed object. In virtual reality conditions (**d**), if the MTP latency is higher than the VOR latency, the projection of the virtual object on the display system will move with the head and will then be perceived as moving. After the MTP latency, the projection of the virtual object is finally compensated (**e**), and the object can be perceived as moving back to its initial position

observed object (in AR) can be perceived as moving (see Fig. 2.6). In summary, knowing the behavior of the VORs can help predicting or alleviating the motion sickness occurrences (Zupan et al. 1994; Adachi et al. 2014).

The vestibulo-ocular reflexes need to be fast: for clear vision, the head movement must be compensated almost immediately; otherwise, it will result in a blurred vision as the one occurring when filming a scene with a moving camera without a stabilization system. To help to reduce the VOR latency, evolution in mankind (and all vertebrates) has resulted in having the three-dimensional orientations of semicircular canal planes highly close to extraocular muscle pulling directions (see Fig. 2.7). In other terms, the eye rotating muscles' pulling directions are almost parallel to corresponding canal planes, thus forming an intrinsic reference frame system. In this system, a "coordinate change" is no longer required to activate or inhibit the eye muscles when the semicircular canals are stimulated. Signals from the semicircular canals are then sent as directly as possible to the eye muscles; the connection involves only three neurons and is correspondingly called the *three-neuron arc* (Szentágothai 1950) (see Fig. 2.8). Using these direct connections, eye movements lag the head movements by less than 10 ms (Aw et al. 1996); hence, the rotational vestibulo-ocular reflex is one of the fastest reflexes in the human body.

The VORs' lag is smaller than MTP latencies measured in HMDs, e.g., >25 ms for the HTC Vive Pro, according to Le Chénéchal and Chatel-Goldman (2018). For

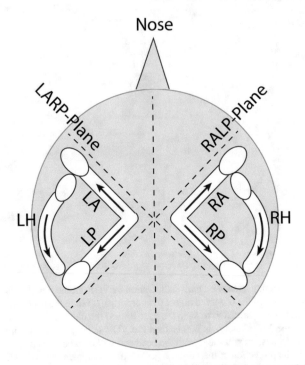

**Fig. 2.7** Orientation of the semicircular canals in the vestibular system. "L/R" stands for "Left/Right", respectively, and "H/A/P" for "Horizontal/Anterior/Posterior". The arrows indicate the direction of the head movement that stimulates the corresponding canal. https://commons. wikimedia.org/wiki/File:Semicircular_Canals.png. Thomas.haslwanter/CC BY-SA (https://creati vecommons.org/licenses/by-sa/3.0)

CAVEs or other virtual reality display setups relying on video projectors, the latency of video projectors alone—namely, without adding latency of head tracking, signal processing, and software calculation, among others—ranges from 15 to 140 ms (Waltemate et al. 2015) and is thus already above VORs' lag. This means that the world instability phenomenon depicted in Fig. 2.1, possibly leading to cybersickness, is barely unavoidable with current technologies.

### 2.2.3.2 Translational VOR

VORs can be distinguished between rotational and translational aspects. When the head rotates (around horizontal, vertical, or torsional axis), the rotational or angular VOR (RVOR), triggered by the semicircular canals, stabilizes distant visual images by rotating the eyes about the same axis but in the opposite direction (Crawford and Vilis 1991). When the head translates, for instance, during walking, the Translational VOR (TVOR), triggered by the otolith organs, maintains the visual fixation point by

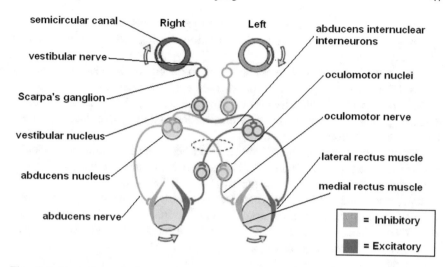

**Fig. 2.8** Illustration of the rotational vestibulo-ocular reflex (RVOR) and the three-neuron arc. https://commons.wikimedia.org/wiki/File:Vestibulo-ocular_reflex.PNG. User:Mikael Häggström/CC BY-SA (http://creativecommons.org/licenses/by-sa/3.0/)

rotating gaze direction in the opposite direction by an amount depending on its distance (Angelaki 2004).

The TVOR also occurs at very short latency (Angelaki and McHenry 1999)—around 10–12 ms—with the same implications on the virtual world's perceived stability as the ones seen before with the RVOR. However, the complexity of the geometrical problem is not as trivial as for the RVOR. Furthermore, no eye movement can result in the stabilization of the whole visual field during translation, as the optic field is not uniform. Hence, the TVOR depends not only on the translation stimulus but also on its direction relative to the head, the orientation of the eyes, and the distance of the fixation point (Schwarz et al. 1989). Distance estimation thus will have a strong impact on translational VOR in VR depending on various VR setup parameters, such as accommodation, vergence, interocular distance, motion parallax, and head tracking (see Chap. 4, Sect. 4.6).

VORs can be characterized by two variables: a gain and a time constant. The gain is the ratio between the amount of eye rotation and the amount of stimulus rotation. Furthermore, the time constant quantifies the time during which the reflex is activated. These two parameters appear to be dependent on the stimulus frequency, as well as highly modifiable and trainable over time to adapt to the situation.

## 2.3 Motion Sickness

Motion sickness is a phenomenon that has been widely studied for years and is still the point of interest of many researchers worldwide. Typical symptoms include cold sweating, belching, retching, pallor, decreased gastric tonus, and typical subjective symptoms such as headache, stomach discomfort, feeling of warmth, nausea, and eventually vomiting.

Early studies of motion sickness date back to the end of the nineteenth century (James 1881; Irwin 1881) with evidence that susceptibility motion sickness may vary between people. For instance, Irwin (1881) and James (1881) found that labyrinthine-defective people, which means people with disorders of the organs of balance in their inner ear, never get sick from motion.

Motion sickness susceptibility may also vary between people with no vestibular deficiencies (Reason and Brand 1975), and questionnaires for motion sickness susceptibility were proposed subsequently (Golding 2006).

It was also found that females do not react the same way as males do against motion sickness for they are more easily sicker than males (Reason and Brand 1975; Dobie et al. 2001; Graeber and Stanney 2002). Gender difference in motion sickness was confirmed in cybersickness in various studies (Viaud-Delmon et al. 1998; Parsons et al. 2004; Tlauka et al. 2005; Ross et al. 2006; Felnhofer et al. 2014; Munafo et al. 2017). Interestingly, cybersickness gender differences were frequently found in space navigation or perception, which may be linked not only with motion sickness but also with cognitive gender differences in spatial navigation (Lawton 1994; Berthoz and Viaud-Delmon 1999; Lambrey and Berthoz 2007), in particular, in using allocentric or egocentric orientation strategies. Indeed, navigation is one of the major actions inducing cybersickness in virtual environments (see Sect. 2.3.5 below and Chap. 4) and thus also one of the major subjects of this book, on which the authors would like to expose a coherent vision of motion sickness in virtual environments.

Independently from gender or physiological considerations, passive persons, such as spectators, get sicker than active persons, as the latter are in control of their motions (Rolnick and Lubow 1991; Stanney and Hash 1998). Typically, drivers do not get sick because they anticipate future movements; therefore, sensed motion is close to what they expect, whereas passengers can easily get sick when they are passive.

The use of immersive technologies such as VR systems or driving simulators leads to a similar phenomenon with the same symptoms (Kolasinski 1995). People in this case often refer to cybersickness or VR sickness rather than motion sickness. Indeed, contrary to motion sickness such as car sickness, being immersed in VR does not necessarily imply that real motion will be perceived and thus be the source of sickness. In fact, in the case of VR, some people also use the term of Visually Induced Motion Sickness (VIMS) to show that sickness is likely to originate from the visual perception of motion from 3D images (Oman 1990; Bos et al. 2008). In driving simulators, however, we will instead use the term of simulator sickness, which may encompass both VIMS and cybersickness.

All these types of sickness may be subcategories of motion sickness (see Fig. 2.9) and in the rest of the book, we will use the term cybersickness or VRISE (Virtual Reality Induced Sickness Effects).

Whatever may be the term used to describe this phenomenon (cybersickness, VR sickness, simulator sickness, VIMS), researchers still do not fully agree on the mechanisms underlying such sensation, and there are still sharp debates on this

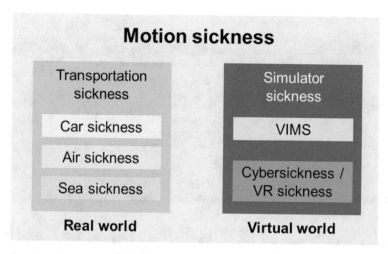

**Fig. 2.9** Motion sickness and its subcategories

issue (see, for example, Kennedy et al. (1993)). In this regard, several theories have tried to explain cybersickness—the most cited being the sensory conflict theory, the ecological theory, and the evolutionary theory.

## 2.3.1 Sensory Conflict

This theory is one of the first to be enounced, in 1975, and is probably now considered as the most relevant to explain cybersickness. Proposed by Reason and Brand, it states that "motion sickness is a self-inflicted maladaptation phenomenon which occurs at the onset and cessation of conditions of sensory rearrangement when the pattern of inputs from the vestibular system, other proprioceptors and vision is at variance with the stored patterns derived from recent transactions with the spatial environment" (Reason and Brand 1975).

In concrete terms, this theory suggests that the orientation of the human body in space mainly depends on the information obtained through four sensory organs: the otoliths that allow sensing linear accelerations and inclination, the semicircular channels that provide information on angular accelerations of the head, the visual system that gives clues on body positions in space, and the proprioceptive system that allows knowing the position of limbs. When a conflict occurs between these organs, sickness arises. In VR and driving simulation, this is, typically, what occurs: when navigating in a virtual environment, we generally do not move physically. Our eyes perceive a movement, but our vestibular system indicates no motion. These two signals conflict with each other in our brain, leading to the so-called cybersickness.

A conceptual model of this process was proposed by Oman (1990). In this model, the body acts as a state system (see Fig. 2.10). Exogenous (externally generated)

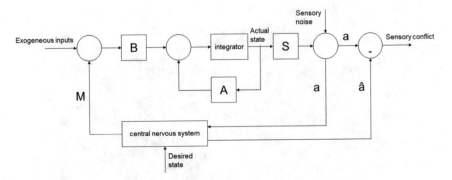

**Fig. 2.10**   Motion sickness model (adapted from Oman (1990))

inputs represent, for example, moving images from a virtual environment. A, B, and S are the state matrices of the body, and a is the resulting actual sensation. The brain, represented by the Central Nervous System (CNS), acts as an observer: from what is perceived (a), it continuously estimates and predicts the body orientation (â) and corrects it through muscles activation (M) to prevent the body from losing balance, for instance. However, if the expected sensation does not match the perceived one, a sensory conflict occurs.

## 2.3.2   Ecological Theory

From Oman's model, we see an interesting feature that relates to motor command. As explained above, the brain tries to continuously correct body orientation. This consideration prefigures a second theory that explains cybersickness, which is called the ecological theory. In fact, arguments were made that the sensory conflict theory cannot completely explain the occurrence of cybersickness from a theoretical point of view, because, on the one hand, considering discrepancies as conflict information instead of something else is just a hypothesis rather than a fact, and on the other hand, there exist many cases that can lead to sensory conflict without inducing cybersickness (Stoffregen and Riccio 1991). Furthermore, the lack of predictive validity of the sensory conflict theory limits its application to the design of virtual environments (Smart et al. 2002). Hence, Riccio and Stoffregen (1991) developed the ecological theory, which relies on postural sway: motion sickness originates from prolonged periods of postural instability. Sensory signals such as visual, auditory, vestibular, and proprioceptive signals from the whole body trigger the body balance function (Kaga 1992). When exposed to 3D visual stimuli, this balance mechanism may not function properly (Takada et al. 2007), which means that the brain struggles in maintaining the body in a fixed upright stance. From this, it was shown that significant increases of postural sway precede motion sickness (Stoffregen et al. 2000), which provides an interesting insight into how to improve the monitoring of motion sickness and thus to prevent it.

### 2.3.3 Evolutionary Theory

The evolutionary theory, introduced by Treisman in 1977 (Treisman 1977), relates motion sickness to intoxication. According to this theory, motion sickness originates from body mechanisms aiming at evacuating toxins present in the stomach. Specifically, motion is viewed as an artificial stimulus that generates a body response initially meant to compensate for the physiological disorders produced by the absorption of toxins. The reason why this theory is qualified as evolutionary is that, according to Treisman, humans do not evolve during their life to adapt to ways of transportation (including cars, trains, airplanes, and boats). To support this assertion, Treisman argues that infants or small children are relatively immune to sickness.

This theory is however highly criticized, as the time needed by a toxin to act on vestibular mechanisms seems too long for emetic reactions to be effective (Harm 2002). Furthermore, emetic reactions are not always observed among cybersick users, which contradicts this theory. Last, regarding Treisman's assertion about the immunity of infants against sickness, past research has shown that this specificity may originate from the immaturity of their spatial orientation mechanisms (Oman 2012).

### 2.3.4 Rest Frame

In addition to the three theories mentioned above, a less known theory is the rest frame theory, formulated by Prothero in 1998 (Prothero 1998), which postulates that humans tend to select things and treat them as stationary references. This idea gets inspiration from physics, where a coordinate system is required to define spatial positions, angular orientations, and motion speeds, providing the observer with a stationary reference called a rest frame. Once stationary and nonstationary references are distinguished, the relative motions of these references are measured by the brain. Therefore, when one is not able to choose an appropriate rest frame, sickness occurs. Specifically, this theory states that cybersickness results from conflicting rest frames caused by the presence of motion cues. Prothero and Parker consider the rest frame as a slight refinement of the sensory conflict theory (Prothero and Parker 2003), which, however, implies focusing on visual stimuli that can influence the selection of rest frames.

## 2.3.5   Factors Affecting Motion Sickness

We already mentioned that cybersickness does not affect individuals in the same way. In fact, cybersickness is a strongly user-dependent phenomenon, and the literature on this aspect is broad (Chang et al. 2020). We then review some of the personal characteristics, as well as technological factors, that are encountered in the occurrence of cybersickness.

### 2.3.5.1   Gender

We introduced differences between males and females as put forward by a robust number of research works (Holmes and Griffin 2001; Hakkinen et al. 2002; Flanagan et al. 2005; Häkkinen et al. 2006; Yang et al. 2012; Jaeger and Mourant 2016; Park et al. 2016). However, some researchers also mention that this difference in gender may arise from a difference in the way self-reports of symptoms, usually done through questionnaires, are completed, as males may under-report their susceptibility to sickness (Biocca 1992). The effect of gender may be occasionally linked to the degree of symptom reporting and the users' willingness to recognize such symptoms under socially controlled psychology; although it is usually admitted that women tend to over-report symptoms compared to men (Ladwig et al. 2000), there exist also works that did not show strong evidence of it regarding motion sickness symptom reporting (Dobie et al. 2001).

Nonetheless, past research found that different reactions between men and women against motion sickness may actually originate from a relationship between hormonal levels and the susceptibility to motion sickness, especially as women have menstrual cycles. For example, women tend to get sick more easily during menstruation (Schwab 1954), and Reason and Brand (1975) added anecdotal evidence of increased sickness during pregnancy. Golding et al. (2005) found that the motion sickness level could fluctuate during the menstrual cycle. For instance, past studies revealed that women not using oral contraceptives reported more severe nausea and sickness symptoms during the peri-menses phase than during the peri-ovulatory phase. In contrast, women using oral contraceptives reported the same level of nausea and sickness symptoms (Matchock et al. 2008).

Another reason explaining differences between genders was found in people's field of view, as women have a wider field of view than that of men (Kennedy and Frank 1985; LaViola 2000). Viaud-Delmon et al. (1998) explain this difference through the sensory conflict theory, arguing that men can better adapt to sensory conflicts than women, which could result in higher sickness in women than in men. In the same vein, Dodgson (2004) examined the human inter-pupillary distance as a sex difference effect and reported that the average inter-pupillary distance for females is around 0.96 times that of males. Read and Bohr (2014) believe that the difference in inter-pupillary distance can affect experiences involving 3D visual stimuli because disparities (i.e., differences in object position on the two retinal images) are restrained by the virtual camera parameters.

### 2.3.5.2  Age

Age is also known to be a parameter affecting motion sickness: the susceptibility to cybersickness follows a Gaussian curve where it grows by age until around 12 and then decreases by age (Kolasinski 1995; Davis et al. 2014).

In practice, this is not that simple, and past research presented contradictory results. In fact, it has been observed that younger generations are less prone to cybersickness than older generations because youngsters are greater users of displays and games since their childhood than the elderly. Being used to visual stimuli present within immersive technologies has a positive effect on the reduction of the occurrence of cybersickness (Stanney and Kennedy 1997; Howarth and Hodder 2008). Hence, people who have a significant gaming experience may be less prone to sickness than non-gamers (George et al. 2014; Rosa et al. 2016), which means that people's own experience may have a strong influence on the susceptibility to cybersickness.

Other studies reported that older people could feel higher dizziness and nausea with 2D stimuli whereas for younger people, greater blurred and double vision, dizziness, and nausea symptoms could be observed with 3D movies, which indicates that older adults are less sensitive to higher vergence demand which is the latent source of blurred and double vision (Yang et al. 2012). Furthermore, due to the loss of accommodation ability, elderly people can experience greater cybersickness symptoms when viewing 2D contents because they have to preserve the same level of vergence or squinting responses. Meanwhile, younger viewers typically have strong accommodation ability to vergence processes, which is more likely to induce side effects when viewing 3D contents (Yang et al. 2012; Read and Bohr 2014).

In a different field, a comparison of age-related differences in driving performance on driving simulators demonstrated that elderly participants (despite being less familiar with computers) are less susceptible to nausea occurring from simulator sickness than other groups of population (Liu et al. 1999).

### 2.3.5.3  Ethnic Origin and Genetic Influences

A deep investigation of the literature reveals relatively little work on the effect of ethnicity on cybersickness. Klosterhalfen et al. (2005) investigate the differences in the susceptibility to motion sickness between Caucasian and Chinese populations. Results indicate that Caucasians are tolerant of rotations for longer periods of time and suffer from less motion sickness than the Chinese. Past research investigates differences from a physiological perspective, with arguments that Chinese people suffer from a greater disturbance in gastric activity than European- and African-American populations, which affects motion sickness susceptibility (Stern et al. 1993).

Independently of ethnic considerations, susceptibility to motion sickness may also originate from hereditary and genetic factors. Yanus and Malmstrom (1994) conducted studies revealing a strong correlation between individuals and their parents in terms of the severity of sickness symptoms. Knox (2014) reported that (1) if both parents are susceptible to motion sickness, their children are five times more susceptible to similar symptoms than other children; (2) 41% of British parents with driving experience also have children susceptible to sickness. Interestingly, monozygotic twins are more prone to motion sickness, with a susceptibility rate around 2.5 times higher than dizygotic twins (Bakwin 1971; Abe et al. 1984; Reavley et al. 2006; Sharma et al. 2008).

Without going deep into genetic aspects, reasons for such an effect of ethnicity and heredity may be found in the peculiarities of some genes. For further detail, we encourage the reader to check the works by Stern et al. (1996), Liu et al. (2002), Finley et al. (2004), Klosterhalfen et al. (2005).

#### 2.3.5.4    Gaming Experience

We have seen that inherent personal characteristics may influence motion sickness susceptibility. However, life experience may also be a significant factor. In particular, with the popularization of video games and the development of immersive video games, research has been done for several years on the influence of gaming experience on motion sickness susceptibility.

Past works mostly agree that gamers are more performant and interact with virtual environments more efficiently than non-gamers, as they develop abilities to achieve rapid and accurate virtual locomotion as well as strong spatial awareness (Smith and Du'Mont 2009), which in turns allows them to suffer from cybersickness much less than non-gamers (Häkkinen et al. 2006; George et al. 2014; Rosa et al. 2016; Dennison et al. 2016; Iskenderova et al. 2017). In particular, people with less computer proficiency, technology, and gaming experience have more of a neutral or negative attitude rather than enthusiasm toward new technology, which may affect their level of stress during a task. Consequently, they pay excessive attention to the sickness symptoms that they experience (Häkkinen et al. 2006).

#### 2.3.5.5    Technological Factors

If individual aspects should be taken into account before immersing people, considerations should also be made from a technological point of view, on which the literature is quite abundant. The field of view (Lin et al. 2002; Sharples et al. 2008), latency (Wilson 2016), low frame rates (LaViola 2000), interfaces (Mestre 2014) and an inappropriate adjustment of interaction parameters (So et al. 2001; Wang et al. 2019), and unsuitable immersive scenario (Lo and So 2001) are factors that commonly influence the level of cybersickness. While their impact has been decreasing thanks to technological progress, they are still significantly perceptible.

#### 2.3.5.6  Motion frequency

Motion sickness experienced by the subject mostly occurs at motion frequencies below 1 Hz (O'Hanlon and McCauley 1973).For instance, it was shown that 0.2 Hz represents a translational oscillation frequency at which motion sickness is maximal (Golding et al. 2001). Higher frequency vibration was shown to be less sickening and may be used to reduce the impact on motion sickness of lower frequencies experienced by the subject (see Chap. 4 Sect. 4.5 and 4.6).

## 2.4  Conclusion

Cybersickness is a highly complex phenomenon that requires deep knowledge of many aspects, from the human visual system to proprioception. Because of its complexity, finding the reasons for its occurrence is still a hot research topic. In particular, the use of immersive technologies combines many factors favoring sickness, which may expose users to intense sickness without any clear ideas on how to alleviate it. Therefore, before considering using immersive technologies extensively, it is essential to know their characteristics in detail, Furthermore, an assessment of software issues is necessary, as well-written and optimized applications with well-described scenarios will help users enjoying immersive technologies. Lastly, as VR experience is user-dependent, it is crucial to fully integrate the user in the design of a VR application.

In Chap. 4, a variety of current methods to get rid of cybersickness will be presented, as well as best practices to develop sickness-free applications.

## References

Abe K, Oda N, Hatta H (1984) Behavioural genetics of early childhood: fears, restlessness, motion sickness and enuresis. Acta Genet Med Gemellol (Roma) 33:303–306. https://doi.org/10.1017/s0001566000007340

Adachi T, Yonekawa T, Fuwamoto Y, Ito S, Iwazaki K, Nagiri S (2014) Simulator motion sickness evaluation based on eye mark recording during vestibulo-ocular reflex. SAE International, Warrendale, PA

Angelaki DE (2004) Eyes on target: what neurons must do for the vestibuloocular reflex during linear motion. J Neurophysiol 92:20–35. https://doi.org/10.1152/jn.00047.2004

Angelaki DE (2009) Vestibulo-ocular reflex. In: Squire LR (ed) Encyclopedia of neuroscience. Academic Press, Oxford, pp 139–146

Angelaki DE, McHenry MQ (1999) Short-latency primate vestibuloocular responses during translation. J Neurophysiol 82:1651–1654. https://doi.org/10.1152/jn.1999.82.3.1651

Aw ST, Halmagyi GM, Haslwanter T, Curthoys IS, Yavor RA, Todd MJ (1996) Three-dimensional vector analysis of the human vestibuloocular reflex in response to high-acceleration head rotations. II. Responses in subjects with unilateral vestibular loss and selective semicircular canal occlusion. J Neurophysiol 76:4021–4030. https://doi.org/10.1152/jn.1996.76.6.4021

Bakwin H (1971) Car-sickness in twins. Dev Med Child Neurol 13:310–312. https://doi.org/10.1111/j.1469-8749.1971.tb03267.x

Bardy BG, Warren WH, Kay BA (1999) The role of central and peripheral vision in postural control duringwalking. Percept Psychophys 61:1356–1368. https://doi.org/10.3758/BF03206186

Bear MF, Connors BW, Paradiso MA (2016) Neurosciences—A la découverte du cerveau, 4e édition. Pradel

Benson AJ, Spencer MB, Stott JR (1986) Thresholds for the detection of the direction of whole-body, linear movement in the horizontal plane. Aviat Space Environ Med 57:1088–1096

Benson AJ, Hutt EC, Brown SF (1989) Thresholds for the perception of whole body angular movement about a vertical axis. Aviat Space Environ Med 60:205–213

Berthoz A (1974) Oculomotricité et proprioception. Revue d'Electroencéphalographie et de Neurophysiologie Clinique 4:569–586. https://doi.org/10.1016/S0370-4475(74)80044-4

Berthoz A (2000) The brain's sense of movement. Harvard University Press

Berthoz A, Viaud-Delmon I (1999) Multisensory integration in spatial orientation. Curr Opin Neurobiol 9:708–712. https://doi.org/10.1016/S0959-4388(99)00041-0

Berthoz A, Pavard B, Young LR (1975) Perception of linear horizontal self-motion induced by peripheral vision (linearvection) basic characteristics and visual-vestibular interactions. Exp Brain Res 23:471–489. https://doi.org/10.1007/BF00234916

Biocca F (1992) Will simulation sickness slow down the diffusion of virtual environment technology? Presence: Teleoper Virtual Environ 1:334–343. https://doi.org/10.1162/pres.1992.1.3.334

Boer ER (1996) Tangent point oriented curve negotiation. In: Proceedings of conference on intelligent vehicles, pp 7–12

Bos JE, Bles W, Groen EL (2008) A theory on visually induced motion sickness. Displays 29:47–57. https://doi.org/10.1016/j.displa.2007.09.002

Bove M, Fenoggio C, Tacchino A, Pelosin E, Schieppati M (2009) Interaction between vision and neck proprioception in the control of stance. Neuroscience 164:1601–1608. https://doi.org/10.1016/j.neuroscience.2009.09.053

Bremmer F, Lappe M (1999) The use of optical velocities for distance discrimination and reproduction during visually simulated self motion. Exp Brain Res 127:33–42

Bringoux L, Schmerber S, Nougier V, Dumas G, Barraud PA, Raphel C (2002) Perception of slow pitch and roll body tilts in bilateral labyrinthine-defective subjects. Neuropsychologia 40:367–372. https://doi.org/10.1016/S0028-3932(01)00103-8

Bruggeman H, Zosh W, Warren WH (2007) Optic flow drives human visuo-locomotor adaptation. Curr Biol 17:2035–2040. https://doi.org/10.1016/j.cub.2007.10.059

Chang E, Kim HT, Yoo B (2020) Virtual reality sickness: a review of causes and measurements. Int J Hum–Comput Interact 0:1–25. https://doi.org/10.1080/10447318.2020.1778351

Clark B, Stewart JD (1968) Comparison of three methods to determine thresholds for perception of angular acceleration. Am J Psychol 81:207–216. https://doi.org/10.2307/1421265

Colombet F, Fang Z, Kemeny A (2015) Pitch tilt rendering for an 8-DOF driving simulator. In: Driving simulation conference 2015 Europe VR, DSC, Tübingen, Germany, pp 55–61

Coutton-Jean C, Mestre DR, Goulon C, Bootsma RJ (2009) The role of edge lines in curve driving. Transport Res Part F: Traffic Psychol Behav 12:483–493. https://doi.org/10.1016/j.trf.2009.04.006

Crawford JD, Vilis T (1991) Axes of eye rotation and Listing's law during rotations of the head. J Neurophysiol 65:407–423. https://doi.org/10.1152/jn.1991.65.3.407

Crowell JA, Banks MS (1993) Perceiving heading with different retinal regions and types of optic flow. Percept Psychophys 53:325–337. https://doi.org/10.3758/BF03205187

Curcio CA, Allen KA (1990) Topography of ganglion cells in human retina. J Comp Neurol 300:5–25. https://doi.org/10.1002/cne.903000103

Davis S, Nesbitt K, Nalivaiko E (2014) A systematic review of cybersickness. In: Proceedings of the 2014 conference on interactive entertainment. Association for Computing Machinery, Newcastle, NSW, Australia, pp 1–9

Dennison MS, Wisti AZ, D'Zmura M (2016) Use of physiological signals to predict cybersickness. Displays 44:42–52. https://doi.org/10.1016/j.displa.2016.07.002

Dichgans J, Brandt T (1978) Visual-vestibular interaction: effects on self-motion perception and postural control. In: Anstis SM, Atkinson J, Blakemore C, Braddick O, Brandt T, Campbell FW, Coren S, Dichgans J, Dodwell PC, Eimas PD, Foley JM, Fox R, Ganz L, Garrett M, Gibson EJ, Girgus JS, Haith MM, Hatwell Y, Hilgard ER, Ingle D, Johansson G, Julesz B, Konishi M, Lackner JR, Levinson E, Liberman AM, Maffei L, Oyama T, Pantle A, Pöppel E, Sekuler R, Stromeyer CF, Studdert-Kennedy M, Teuber H-L, Yin RK, Held R, Leibowitz HW, Teuber H-L (eds) Perception. Springer, Berlin, Heidelberg, pp 755–804

Dobie T, McBride D, Dobie T, May J (2001) The effects of age and sex on susceptibility to motion sickness. Aviat Space Environ Med 72:13–20

Dodgson NA (2004) Variation and extrema of human interpupillary distance. In: Merritt JO, Benton SA, Bolas MT (eds) Woods AJ. San Jose, CA, pp 36–46

Enroth-Cugell C, Robson JG (1984) Functional characteristics and diversity of cat retinal ganglion cells. Basic characteristics and quantitative description. Invest Ophthalmol Vis Sci 25:250–267

Fang Z, Colombet F, Collinet J-C, Kemeny A (2014) Roll tilt thresholds for 8 DOF driving simulators. In: Proceedings of the driving simulation conference 2014 Europe, Paris, France

Felnhofer A, Kothgassner OD, Hauk N, Beutl L, Hlavacs H, Kryspin-Exner I (2014) Physical and social presence in collaborative virtual environments: exploring age and gender differences with respect to empathy. Comput Hum Behav 31:272–279. https://doi.org/10.1016/j.chb.2013.10.045

Finley JC, O'Leary M, Wester D, MacKenzie S, Shepard N, Farrow S, Lockette W (2004) A genetic polymorphism of the alpha2-adrenergic receptor increases autonomic responses to stress. J Appl Physiol 96:2231–2239. https://doi.org/10.1152/japplphysiol.00527.2003

Fisher SK, Ciuffreda KJ (1988) Accommodation and apparent distance. Perception 17:609–621. https://doi.org/10.1068/p170609

Flanagan MB, May JG, Dobie TG (2005) Sex differences in tolerance to visually-induced motion sickness. Aviat Space Environ Med 76:642–646

George P, Kemeny A, Colombet F, Merienne F, Chardonnet J-R, Thouvenin IM (2014) Evaluation of smartphone-based interaction techniques in a CAVE in the context of immersive digital project review. In: The engineering reality of virtual reality 2014. International Society for Optics and Photonics, p 901203

Gianna C, Heimbrand S, Gresty M (1996) Thresholds for detection of motion direction during passive lateral whole-body acceleration in normal subjects and patients with bilateral loss of labyrinthine function. Brain Res Bull 40:443–447. https://doi.org/10.1016/0361-9230(96)00140-2

Gibson JJ (1979) The ecological approach to visual perception. Psychology Press

Golding JF (2006) Predicting individual differences in motion sickness susceptibility by questionnaire. Pers Individ Differ 41:237–248. https://doi.org/10.1016/j.paid.2006.01.012

Golding JF, Kadzere P, Gresty MA (2005) Motion sickness susceptibility fluctuates through the menstrual cycle. Aviat Space Environ Med 76:970–973

Golding JF, Phil D, Mueller AG, Gresty MA (2001) A motion sickness maximum around the 0.2 hz frequency range of horizontal translational oscillation. Aviat Space Environ Med 72:188–192

Graeber DA, Stanney KM (2002) Gender differences in visually induced motion sickness. In: Proceedings of the human factors and ergonomics society annual meeting, vol 46, pp 2109–2113. https://doi.org/10.1177/154193120204602602

Graf W, Klam F (2006) Le système vestibulaire: anatomie fonctionnelle et comparée, évolution et développement. CR Palevol 5:637–655. https://doi.org/10.1016/j.crpv.2005.12.009

Grant VW (1942) Accommodation and convergence in visual space perception. J Exp Psychol 31:89–104. https://doi.org/10.1037/h0062359

Gray R, Regan D (2000) Simulated self-motion alters perceived time to collision. Curr Biol 10:587–590

Groen EL, Bles W (2004) How to use body tilt for the simulation of linear self motion. J Vestib Res 14:375–385

Groen EL, Howard IP, Cheung BSK (1999) Influence of body roll on visually induced sensations of self-tilt and rotation. Perception 28:287–297. https://doi.org/10.1068/p2850

Hagner D, Webster JG (1988) Telepresence for touch and proprioception in teleoperator systems. IEEE Trans Syst Man Cybern. https://doi.org/10.1109/21.23102

Hakkinen J, Vuori T, Paakka M (2002) Postural stability and sickness symptoms after HMD use. In: IEEE International conference on systems, man and cybernetics, pp 147–152

Häkkinen J, Liinasuo M, Takatalo J, Nyman G (2006) Visual comfort with mobile stereoscopic gaming. In: Stereoscopic displays and virtual reality systems XIII. International Society for Optics and Photonics, p 60550A

Hamann C, Schönfeld U, Clarke AH (2001) Otolith-ocular reflex in linear acceleration of low frequencies. HNO 49:818–824. https://doi.org/10.1007/s001060170030

Harm DL (2002) Motion sickness neurophysiology, physiological correlates, and treatment. In: Handbook of virtual environments. CRC Press, pp 677–702

Heerspink H, Berkouwer W, Stroosma O, van Paassen R, Mulder M, Mulder B (2005) Evaluation of vestibular thresholds for motion detection in the SIMONA research simulator. In: AIAA modeling and simulation technologies conference and exhibit. American Institute of Aeronautics and Astronautics

Hettinger LJ, Berbaum KS, Kennedy RS, Dunlap WP, Nolan MD (1990) Vection and simulator sickness. Mil Psychol 2:171–181. https://doi.org/10.1207/s15327876mp0203_4

Holmes SR, Griffin MJ (2001) Correlation between heart rate and the severity of motion sickness caused by optokinetic stimulation. J Psychophysiol 15:35–42. https://doi.org/10.1027//0269-8803.15.1.35

Howarth PA, Hodder SG (2008) Characteristics of habituation to motion in a virtual environment. Displays 29:117–123. https://doi.org/10.1016/j.displa.2007.09.009

Irwin JA (1881) The pathology of sea-sickness. Lancet 118:907–909. https://doi.org/10.1016/S0140-6736(02)38129-7

Iskenderova A, Weidner F, Broll W (2017) Drunk virtual reality gaming: exploring the influence of alcohol on cybersickness. In: Proceedings of the annual symposium on computer-human interaction in play. Association for Computing Machinery, Amsterdam, The Netherlands, pp 561–572

Jaeger BK, Mourant RR (2016) Comparison of simulator sickness using static and dynamic walking simulators. In: Proceedings of the human factors and ergonomics society annual meeting. https://doi.org/10.1177/154193120104502709

James W (1881) Sense of dizziness in deaf-mutes. Mind 412–413. https://doi.org/10.1093/mind/os-VI.23.412

Kaga K (1992) Memaino Kouzo: structure of vertigo. Kanehara Shuppan Co 1:23–26

Kaplan E, Bernadete E (2001) The dynamics of primate retinal ganglion cells. In: Progress in brain research. Gulf Professional Publishing

Kennedy RS, Frank LH (1985) A review of motion sickness with special reference to simulator sickness. Canyon Research Group Inc

Kennedy RS, Lane NE, Berbaum KS, Lilienthal MG (1993) Simulator sickness questionnaire: an enhanced method for quantifying simulator sickness. Int J Aviat Psychol 3:203–220. https://doi.org/10.1207/s15327108ijap0303_3

Klosterhalfen S, Kellermann S, Pan F, Stockhorst U, Hall G, Enck P (2005) Effects of ethnicity and gender on motion sickness susceptibility. Aviat Space Environ Med 76:1051–1057

Knox GW (2014) Motion sickness: an evolutionary and genetic basis for the negative reinforcement model. Aviat Space Environ Med 85:46–49. https://doi.org/10.3357/asem.3519.2014

Kolasinski EM (1995) Simulator sickness in virtual environments. U.S. Army Research Institute for the Behavioral and Social Sciences

Ladwig K-H, Marten-Mittag B, Formanek B, Dammann G (2000) Gender differences of symptom reporting and medical health care utilization in the German population. Eur J Epidemiol 16:511–518

Lambrey S, Berthoz A (2007) Gender differences in the use of external landmarks versus spatial representations updated by self-motion. J Integr Neurosci 06:379–401. https://doi.org/10.1142/S021963520700157X

Land MF, Lee DN (1994) Where we look when we steer. Nature 369:742–744. https://doi.org/10.1038/369742a0

Lappe M, Bremmer F, van den Berg AV (1999) Perception of self-motion from visual flow. Trends Cognit Sci 3:329–336. https://doi.org/10.1016/S1364-6613(99)01364-9

LaViola JJ (2000) A discussion of cybersickness in virtual environments. SIGCHI Bull 32:47–56

Lawton CA (1994) Gender differences in way-finding strategies: relationship to spatial ability and spatial anxiety. Sex Roles 30:765–779. https://doi.org/10.1007/BF01544230

Le Chénéchal M, Chatel-Goldman J (2018) HTC Vive Pro time performance benchmark for scientific research. In: ICAT-EGVE 2018. Limassol, Cyprus

Lee DN (1980) The optic flow field: the foundation of vision. Philos Trans R Soc Lond B Biol Sci 290:169–179

Lee DN, Bootsma RJ, Land M, Regan D, Gray R (2009) Lee's 1976 paper. Perception 38:837–858

Li L, Warren WH (2002) Retinal flow is sufficient for steering during observer rotation. Psychol Sci 13:485–490. https://doi.org/10.1111/1467-9280.00486

Lin JJ-W, Duh HBL, Parker DE, Abi-Rached H, Furness TA (2002) Effects of field of view on presence, enjoyment, memory, and simulator sickness in a virtual environment. Proc IEEE Virtual Real 2002:164–171

Liu L, Miyazaki M, Watson B (1999) Norms and validity of the DriVR: a virtual reality driving assessment for persons with head injuries. Cyberpsychol Behav 2:53–67. https://doi.org/10.1089/cpb.1999.2.53

Liu L, Yuan L, Wang HB, Yu LS, Zheng J, Luo CQ, Wang Y (2002) The human alpha(2A)-AR gene and the genotype of site-1296 and the susceptibility to motion sickness. Sheng Wu Hua Xue Yu Sheng Wu Wu Li Xue Bao 34:291–297

Lo WT, So RHY (2001) Cybersickness in the presence of scene rotational movements along different axes. Appl Ergon 32:1–14. https://doi.org/10.1016/S0003-6870(00)00059-4

Matchock RL, Levine ME, Gianaros PJ, Stern RM (2008) Susceptibility to Nausea and motion sickness as a function of the menstrual cycle. Women's Health Iss 18:328–335. https://doi.org/10.1016/j.whi.2008.01.006

Mestre DR (2014) Evaluation of navigation interfaces in virtual environments. In: The engineering reality of virtual reality 2014. International Society for Optics and Photonics, p 901207

Munafo J, Diedrick M, Stoffregen TA (2017) The virtual reality head-mounted display Oculus Rift induces motion sickness and is sexist in its effects. Exp Brain Res 235:889–901

Nesti A, Masone C, Barnett-Cowan M, Robuffo Giordano P, Bülthoff HH, Pretto P (2012) Roll rate thresholds and perceived realism in driving simulation. In: Proceedings of the driving simulation conference 2012 Europe, Paris, France

O'Hanlon JF, McCauley ME (1973) Motion sickness incidence as a function of the frequency and acceleration of vertical sinusoidal motion. Aerospace Medicine 45:366–369

Oman CM (1990) Motion sickness: a synthesis and evaluation of the sensory conflict theory. Can J Physiol Pharmacol 68:294–303. https://doi.org/10.1139/y90-044

Oman CM (2012) Are evolutionary hypotheses for motion sickness "just-so" stories? J Vestib Res 22:117–127. https://doi.org/10.3233/VES-2011-0432

Palmisano S, Chan AYC (2004) Jitter and size effects on vection are immune to experimental instructions and demands. Perception 33:987–1000. https://doi.org/10.1068/p5242

Park GD, Allen RW, Fiorentino D, Rosenthal TJ, Cook ML (2016) Simulator sickness scores according to symptom susceptibility, age, and gender for an older driver assessment study. In: Proceedings of the human factors and ergonomics society annual meeting. https://doi.org/10.1177/154193120605002607

Parsons TD, Larson P, Kratz K, Thiebaux M, Bluestein B, Buckwalter JG, Rizzo AA (2004) Sex differences in mental rotation and spatial rotation in a virtual environment. Neuropsychologia 42:555–562. https://doi.org/10.1016/j.neuropsychologia.2003.08.014

Pavard B, Berthoz A (1977) Linear acceleration modifies the perceived velocity of a moving visual scene. Perception 6:529–540. https://doi.org/10.1068/p060529

Post RB (1988) Circular vection is independent of stimulus eccentricity. Perception 17:737–744. https://doi.org/10.1068/p170737

Pretto P, Nesti A, Nooij S, Losert M, Bülthoff HH (2014) Variable roll-rate perception in driving simulation. In: Proceedings of the driving simulation conference 2014 Europe, Paris, France

Prothero JD (1998) The role of rest frames in vection, presence and motion sickness. PhD thesis, University of Washington, HIT-Lab

Prothero J, Parker D (2003) A unified approach to presence and motion sickness. Virtual and adaptive environments: applications, implications, and human performance issues, pp 47–66. https://doi.org/10.1201/9781410608888.ch3

Read JCA, Bohr I (2014) User experience while viewing stereoscopic 3D television. Ergonomics 57:1140–1153. https://doi.org/10.1080/00140139.2014.914581

Reason JT, Brand JJ (1975) Motion sickness. Academic Press, Oxford, England

Reavley CM, Golding JF, Cherkas LF, Spector TD, MacGregor AJ (2006) Genetic influences on motion sickness susceptibility in adult women: a classical twin study. Aviat Space Environ Med 77:1148–1152

Redlick FP, Jenkin M, Harris LR (2001) Humans can use optic flow to estimate distance of travel. Vision Res 41:213–219. https://doi.org/10.1016/S0042-6989(00)00243-1

Remington LA (2012) Clinical anatomy and physiology of the visual system. Elsevier

Reymond G, Kemeny A, Droulez J, Berthoz A (2001) Role of lateral acceleration in curve driving: Driver model and experiments on a real vehicle and a driving simulator. Hum Factors 43:483–495. https://doi.org/10.1518/001872001775898188

Riccio GE, Stoffregen TA (1991) An ecological theory of motion sickness and postural instability. Ecol Psychol 3:195–240. https://doi.org/10.1207/s15326969eco0303_2

Riecke BE, Schulte-Pelkum J, Avraamides MN, Heyde MVD, Bülthoff HH (2006) Cognitive factors can influence self-motion perception (vection) in virtual reality. ACM Trans Appl Percept 3:194–216. https://doi.org/10.1145/1166087.1166091

Rodenburg M, Stassen HPW, Maas AJJ (1981) The threshold of perception of angular acceleration as a function of duration. Biol Cybern 39:223–226. https://doi.org/10.1007/BF00342774

Rolnick A, Lubow RE (1991) Why is the driver rarely motion sick? The role of controllability in motion sickness. Ergonomics 34:867–879. https://doi.org/10.1080/00140139108964831

Rosa PJ, Morais D, Gamito P, Oliveira J, Saraiva T (2016) The immersive virtual reality experience: a typology of users revealed through multiple correspondence analysis combined with cluster analysis technique. Cyberpsychol Behav Soc Netw 19:209–216. https://doi.org/10.1089/cyber.2015.0130

Ross SP, Skelton RW, Mueller SC (2006) Gender differences in spatial navigation in virtual space: implications when using virtual environments in instruction and assessment. Virtual Real 10:175–184. https://doi.org/10.1007/s10055-006-0041-7

Schwab RS (1954) The nonlabyrinthine causes of motion sickness. Int Rec Med Gen Pract Clin 167:631–637

Schwarz U, Busettini C, Miles F (1989) Ocular responses to linear motion are inversely proportional to viewing distance. Science 245:1394. https://doi.org/10.1126/science.2506641

Sharma K, Sharma P, Sharma A, Singh G (2008) Phenylthiocarbamide taste perception and susceptibility to motion sickness: linking higher susceptibility with higher phenylthiocarbamide taste acuity. J Laryngol Otol 122:1064–1073. https://doi.org/10.1017/S0022215107001442

Sharples S, Cobb S, Moody A, Wilson JR (2008) Virtual reality induced symptoms and effects (VRISE): comparison of head mounted display (HMD), desktop and projection display systems. Displays 29:58–69. https://doi.org/10.1016/j.displa.2007.09.005

Shibata T, Kim J, Hoffman DM, Banks MS (2011) Visual discomfort with stereo displays: effects of viewing distance and direction of vergence-accommodation conflict. In: Stereoscopic displays and applications XXII. International Society for Optics and Photonics, p 78630P

Smart LJ, Stoffregen TA, Bardy BG (2002) Visually induced motion sickness predicted by postural instability. Hum Factors 44:451–465. https://doi.org/10.1518/0018720024497745

Smith SP, Du'Mont S (2009) Measuring the effect of gaming experience on virtual environment navigation tasks. In: 2009 IEEE symposium on 3D user interfaces, pp 3–10

So RHY, Lo WT, Ho ATK (2001) Effects of navigation speed on motion sickness caused by an immersive virtual environment. Hum Factors 43:452–461. https://doi.org/10.1518/001872001775898223

Sousa ASP, Silva A, Tavares JMRS (2012) Biomechanical and neurophysiological mechanisms related to postural control and efficiency of movement: a review. Somatosens Mot Res 29:131–143. https://doi.org/10.3109/08990220.2012.725680

Stanney KM, Hash P (1998) Locus of user-initiated control in virtual environments: influences on cybersickness. Presence: Teleoper Virtual Environ 7:447–459. https://doi.org/10.1162/105474698565848

Stanney KM, Kennedy RS (1997) The psychometrics of cybersickness. Commun ACM 40:66–69

Stern RM, Hu S, LeBlanc R, Koch KL (1993) Chinese hyper-susceptibility to vection-induced motion sickness. Aviat Space Environ Med 64:827–830

Stern RM, Hu S, Uijtdehaage SH, Muth E, Xu LH, Koch KL (1996) Asian hypersusceptibility to motion sickness. Hum Hered. https://doi.org/10.1159/000154318

Stoffregen TA, Riccio GE (1991) An ecological critique of the sensory conflict theory of motion sickness. Ecol Psychol 3:159–194. https://doi.org/10.1207/s15326969eco0303_1

Stoffregen TA, Hettinger LJ, Haas MW, Roe MM, Smart LJ (2000) Postural instability and motion sickness in a fixed-base flight simulator. Hum Factors 42:458–469. https://doi.org/10.1518/001872000779698097

Strasburger H, Rentschler I, Jüttner M (2011) Peripheral vision and pattern recognition: a review. J Vis 11:13–13. https://doi.org/10.1167/11.5.13

Szentágothai J (1950) The elementary vestibulo-ocular reflex arc. J Neurophysiol 13:395–407. https://doi.org/10.1152/jn.1950.13.6.395

Takada H, Fujitake K, Miyao M, Matsuura Y (2007) Indices to detect visually induced motion sickness using stabilometry. In: First international symposium on visually induced motion sickness, fatigue, and photosensitive epileptic seizures (VIMS2007), pp 178–183

Tarita-Nistor L, González EG, Spigelman AJ, Steinbach MJ (2006) Linear vection as a function of stimulus eccentricity, visual angle, and fixation. J Vestib Res 16:265–272

Taylor CJ, Košecká J, Blasi R, Malik J (1999) A comparative study of vision-based lateral control strategies for autonomous highway driving. Int J Robot Res 18:442–453. https://doi.org/10.1177/027836499901800502

Tlauka M, Brolese A, Pomeroy D, Hobbs W (2005) Gender differences in spatial knowledge acquired through simulated exploration of a virtual shopping centre. J Environ Psychol 25:111–118. https://doi.org/10.1016/j.jenvp.2004.12.002

Treisman M (1977) Motion sickness: an evolutionary hypothesis. Science 197:493–495. https://doi.org/10.1126/science.301659

Tresilian JR (1995) Perceptual and cognitive processes in time-to-contact estimation: Analysis of prediction-motion and relative judgment tasks. Percept Psychophys 57:231–245

Tuthill JC, Azim E (2018) Proprioception. Curr Biol 28:R194–R203. https://doi.org/10.1016/j.cub.2018.01.064

van Beers RJ, Sittig AC, van der Gon JJD (1999) Integration of proprioceptive and visual position-information: an experimentally supported model. J Neurophysiol 81:1355–1364. https://doi.org/10.1152/jn.1999.81.3.1355

van Egmond AAJ, Groen JJ, Jongkees LBW (1949) The mechanics of the semicircular canal. J Physiol 110:1–17. https://doi.org/10.1113/jphysiol.1949.sp004416

Viaud-Delmon I, Ivanenko YP, Berthoz A, Jouvent R (1998) Sex, lies and virtual reality. Nat Neurosci 1:15–16. https://doi.org/10.1038/215

Von Hofsten C (1976) The role of convergence in visual space perception. Vis Res 16:193–198. https://doi.org/10.1016/0042-6989(76)90098-5

Waltemate T, Hülsmann F, Pfeiffer T, Kopp S, Botsch M (2015) Realizing a low-latency virtual reality environment for motor learning. In: Proceedings of the 21st ACM symposium on virtual reality software and technology. Association for Computing Machinery, Beijing, China, pp 139–147

Wang Y, Chardonnet J-R, Merienne F (2019) Design of a semiautomatic travel technique in VR environments. In: 2019 IEEE conference on virtual reality and 3D user interfaces (VR), pp 1223–1224

Wann J, Land M (2000) Steering with or without the flow: is the retrieval of heading necessary? Trends Cognit Sci 4:319–324. https://doi.org/10.1016/S1364-6613(00)01513-8

Warren WH, Hannon DJ (1988) Direction of self-motion is perceived from optical flow. Nature 336:162–163

Warren WH, Kurtz KJ (1992) The role of central and peripheral vision in perceiving the direction of self-motion. Percept Psychophys 51:443–454. https://doi.org/10.3758/BF03211640

Warren WH, Morris MW, Kalish M (1988) Perception of translational heading from optical flow. J Exp Psychol Hum Percept Perform 14:646

Watanabe M, Rodieck RW (1989) Parasol and midget ganglion cells of the primate retina. J Comp Neurol 289:434–454. https://doi.org/10.1002/cne.902890308

Wentink M, Bos J, Groen E, Hosman R (2006) Development of the motion perception toolbox. In: AIAA modeling and simulation technologies conference and exhibit. American Institute of Aeronautics and Astronautics

Wilson M (2016) The effect of varying latency in a head-mounted display on task performance and motion sickness. PhD thesis, Clemson University

Wright WG, DiZio P, Lackner JR (2006) Perceived self-motion in two visual contexts: dissociable mechanisms underlie perception. J Vestib Res 16:23–28

Yang S, Schlieski T, Selmins B, Cooper S, Doherty R, Corriveau P, Sheedy J (2012) Stereoscopic viewing and reported perceived immersion and symptoms. Optom Vis Sci 89:1068–1080. https://doi.org/10.1097/OPX.0b013e31825da430

Yanus TM, Malmstrom FV (1994) Is motion sickness hereditary? In: Proceedings of the human factors and ergonomics society annual meeting, vol 38, pp 796–800. https://doi.org/10.1177/154193129403801304

Zhao J, Allison RS, Vinnikov M, Jennings S (2017) Estimating the motion-to-photon latency in head mounted displays. In: 2017 IEEE virtual reality (VR), pp 313–314

Zupan L, Droulez J, Darlot C, Denise P, Maruani A (1994) Modelization of vestibulo-ocular reflex (VOR) and motion sickness prediction. In: Marinaro M, Morasso PG (eds) ICANN '94. Springer, London, pp 106–109

# Chapter 3
# Visualization and Motion Systems

**Abstract** This section provides a description of visualization and motion rendering systems used for virtual systems and simulators. The characteristics of visual systems, such as image resolution, brightness, contrast, and frequency, have a substantial impact on immersion, and display latency may induce severe cybersickness. A brief history of HMDs illustrates the evolution of virtual visualization systems, which are currently experiencing a renewed interest. A special focus is given to passive and active stereoscopic rendering, including autostereoscopic systems with a short survey on light field technology. The latter makes 3D vision possible without the use of specific polarization or active glasses, although at the price of increased system complexity and installation costs. Motion systems include various devices. Affordable and compact vibration systems provide face value and generic motion. Treadmills allow to extend natural walking. High-performance motion rendering systems include 6-axis and/or linear actuators, reproducing human motion perception and avoiding visuo-vestibular conflicts. Tilt coordination—a motion rendering technique for sustained accelerations, based on the gravito-inertial equivalence—is presented. The chapter completes this overview with a presentation of the main Motion Cueing Algorithms (MCA) for motion rendering—from classical and adaptive cueing approaches to prediction-based Model Predictive Control (MPC) techniques.

## 3.1 Visualization Systems

### 3.1.1 Display Systems

#### 3.1.1.1 Main Characteristics

Display systems used in simulation and Virtual Reality can significantly vary in terms of technology, characteristics, performances, and price. Most systems are either based on video projectors or electric visual displays commonly called screens (including television sets, smartphone screens, and computer monitors). Knowing the main

A. Kemeny et al., *Getting Rid of Cybersickness*,
https://doi.org/10.1007/978-3-030-59342-1_3

advantages and drawbacks of these two technologies can thus be very helpful to determine their potential impacts on the image perceived by the driver and the potentially resulting cybersickness.

Some characteristics, such as resolution, luminance, refresh frequency, and latency, are shared by both video projectors and screens. The resolution is the number of pixels that a screen or a video projector can display. For example, the "Full High Definition (FHD)" resolution corresponds to 1920 × 1080 pixels and the "4 K Ultra High Definition (4 K UHD)" to 3840 × 2160 pixels. The resolution should not be confused with pixel density, corresponding to the number of pixels per distance unit (e.g., pixels per inch, or PPI). For example, a TV and a smartphone may have the same resolution, but the smartphone screen will have a higher pixel density because it is smaller than the TV screen. Depending on the distance from which the user is viewing the displayed image, the image resolution must be put in parallel to human eye angular resolution (1 arc min for 6/6 acuity according to EN ISO 8596). As an example, to match this human eye angular resolution, a 2 m wide screen seen from a 2 meters distance should have a minimum horizontal resolution of 3438 pixels (see Fig. 3.1). Using a 4 K image (3840 × 2160) is sufficient in this first example. If the screen is 3 meters wide, the minimum horizontal resolution becomes 5157 pixels and an 8 K image (7680 × 4320) is thus necessary to match the human eye's angular resolution.

The luminance is relative to the quantity of light emitted by the display system and is expressed in candelas per square meter (cd/m$^2$). For video projectors, a value in lumens is commonly used, as the luminance of the displayed image depends on

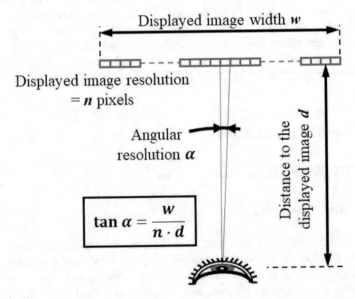

**Fig. 3.1** Relation between the resolution $n$ of a displayed image and the angular resolution $\alpha$, as a function of the image width $w$ and the distance to the displayed image $d$

its distance to the video projector and the characteristics of the projection surface. Luminance is sometimes abusively called brightness but should not be confused with it, as brightness is the subjective impression of the objective luminance. Luminance in the real world can achieve much higher values than display systems, such as $1.6 \times 10^9$ cd/m$^2$ for the sun at noon[1] against 50–300 cd/m$^2$ for typical computer displays.

Refresh frequency or refresh rate is the number of times in a second that the display system updates its buffer, and is not to be confused with the frame rate, which refers to the video source (the software's output). Display systems latency corresponds to the display lag between the time of the signal input and the time this input is displayed on the screen, and it includes not only the pixel response time but also the complete internal processing of the system. However, it does not include additional delays due to acquisition, software processing, and signal routing, among others. The complete overall latency between the user's actual motion or action and the resulting update on the visual display is called the Motion To Photon (MTP) latency (Zhao et al. 2017), as anticipated in Chap. 2, Sect. 2.2.3.

### 3.1.1.2  Screens

Different technologies exist for electric visual displays or standard screens (see Table 3.1). The first technology used were Cathode-Ray Tubes (CRTs), composed of a vacuum tube in which one or more electron guns send electron beams on a phosphorescent screen to create an image. This technology is almost no longer in use and thus will not be further detailed here.

One of the most widespread screen technologies over the past few decades are Liquid-Crystal Displays (LCDs)—flat-panel displays using properties of liquid crystals combined with polarizers to block or let light pass from a backlight. Liquid crystals are arranged in a matrix shape to create the pixels and do not emit light by themselves—they let it pass through a certain amount of the backlight depending on the voltage applied across them. Compared to CRT displays, LCD screens are thinner and less heavy, have a low power consumption (and thus little heat emitted during operation), and no geometric distortion, among other advantages. Furthermore, they can be made in almost any size and resolution, which, in the past few decades, has made the rise of transportable displays in portable PCs and smartphones, and then in public and affordable VR helmets, possible (see Sect. 3.1.2, "A brief history of HMDs").

Organic Light-Emitting Diode (OLED, or organic LED) screens are composed of a matrix of LEDs in which the emissive electroluminescent layer is a film of organic compound emitting light in response to an electric current. OLED (or AMOLED for active-matrix OLED) are progressively replacing LCD screens in smartphones

---

[1]Lighting Design and Simulation Knowledge base—Lighting Design Glossary—Luminance. https://www.schorsch.com/en/kbase/glossary/luminance.html.

**Table 3.1** Summary of the main characteristics of LCD, OLED, and microLED screen technologies

|                                      | LCD                                    | OLED                                                          | MicroLED                                                                                           |
| ------------------------------------ | -------------------------------------- | ------------------------------------------------------------ | ------------------------------------------------------------------------------------------------- |
| Maximum resolution                   | 8 K (7680 × 4320)                      | 8 K (7680 × 4320)                                            | 16 K and virtually infinite as microLED units can be juxtaposed without visible borders[2]        |
| Definition (minimum pixel size)      | <0.040 mm                              | <0.040 mm                                                    | 0.9 mm                                                                                             |
| Brightness/luminance                 | Around 500 cd/m$^2$ [3]                | Around 150 cd/m$^2$ for full-screen white [4]               | 1000 cd/m$^2$                                                                                      |
| Contrast                             | /                                      | Virtually infinite as LEDs emit no light with black         | Virtually infinite as LEDs emit no light with black                                               |
| Refreshfrequency                     | Up to 240 Hz for gamer gaming monitors | 120 Hz[5]                                                    | 120 Hz[6]                                                                                          |
| Latency                              | Between 1 and 8 ms                     | Under 0.1 ms[7]                                              | Probably identical to OLED but no objective measure is available yet                              |
| Maximum diagonal size                | Up to 108″ (2.78 m)[8]                 | Up to 88″ (2.24 m) [9]                                      | Virtually infinite as microLED units can be juxtaposed without visible borders                   |

(e.g., Samsung Galaxy S20[10] and Apple iPhone 11 Pro[11]), portable computers, TV screens, and VR headsets (e.g., Oculus Quest [12], HTC Vive Pro[13], and PlayStation VR[14]). Compared to LCD screens, they can be thinner and lighter due to the non-necessity of a backlight, as LEDs emit light directly. For VR headsets, this weight gain is crucial for the user's comfort and "natural" behavior: the lower the weight added on the user's head, the less inertia is added to the head with possible impact on the head's motion behavior. As there is no backlight, the contrast is also enhanced and is virtually infinite as there is no light emitted when displaying black color. LCD screens indeed still emit a small amount of light when displaying black, as the crystals are not able to block all the backlight. Among other advantages, OLED screens can

---

[10] Samsung Galaxy S20: https://www.samsung.com/us/mobile/galaxy-s20-5g/design/.

[11] Apple iPhone 11 Pro: https://www.apple.com/iphone-11-pro/.

[12] Oculus Device Specifications: https://developer.oculus.com/design/oculus-device-specs/.

[13] HTC Vive Pro: https://enterprise.vive.com/us/product/vive-pro/.

[14] PlayStation VR: https://www.playstation.com/en-gb/explore/playstation-vr/tech-specs/.

also be flexible[15] and transparent,[16] the latter offering an interesting potential for Augmented Reality.

MicroLED (also known as mLED or μLED) is an emerging technology somewhat similar to OLED screens, consisting of an array of emissive materials forming the pixel elements, but with inorganic LEDs. Conventional LED technology keeps the advantages of OLED screens while also offering a higher total brightness (up to 1000 cd/m$^2$ [17]) as well as less power consumption. MicroLEDs are still expensive and not yet ready for mass production but have a huge potential to replace video projectors for CAVE or simulator installations in the future, like at Mitsubishi Motors, to give an example[18].

The difficulty to define a coherent product with all of the necessary VR characteristics is well illustrated with the advent of 3D televisions, displaying stereoscopic images with dedicated glasses, active-shuttering filtering (see *Stereoscopy* section below), since the beginning of the 2010s. The lack of content, the requirement for viewers to wear 3D glasses, calibration issues, but also the lack of motion parallax (Chap. 1, Sect. 1.4.1) caused that it never really took off as expected,[19] and production was halted in 2016.

### 3.1.1.3 Video Projectors

A video projector projects an image corresponding to the received video signal by using a lens system. The image perceived by the user depends not only on the video projector characteristics but also on the projection screen's size, distance, color, and surface. Hence, the projection screen's gain—namely, the ratio between the incident and reflected light—has to be selected to achieve the best compromise between reflected brightness and contrast.

Video projectors are designed to project on a flat surface perpendicular to the optical axis of the video projector. When the projection screen of the visualization system is not as described before like, for example, with cylindrical or spherical screens, the projected image is distorted. It has then to be compensated both in geometry and in luminosity as all the pixels are not at the same distance from the video projector. This image treatment is added to the total latency between image computing and image displaying. This latency increase may lead to cybersickness (see Chap. 4, Sect. 4.6).

---

[15]OLED-info, Flexible OLEDs: introduction and market status, 2019: https://www.oled-info.com/flexible-oled.

[16]OLED-info, Transparent OLEDs: introduction and market status, 2019: https://www.oled-info.com/transparent-oleds.

[17]Sony Crystal LED: https://pro.sony/technology/crystal-led.

[18]Sony Crystal LED transforms vehicle design at Mitsubishi Motors: https://pro.sony/technology/crystal-led/mitsubishi-cled.

[19]Independent, 3D TV is dead, 2017-01-25: https://www.independent.co.uk/life-style/gadgets-and-tech/news/3d-tv-dead-last-manufacturers-lg-sony-give-up-tech-trend-glasses-home-cinema-television-a7546091.html.

Projection technologies vary. The first (analogic) video projectors used CRT technology identical to CRT screens, which is now obsolete; hence, it will not be further detailed here. The first digital video projectors used LCD technology (Dolgoff 1991): a light source was emitted through an LCD, and a lens system was used to project the image. In more recent systems, known as tri-LCDs, the light source is split into three primary colors before going through three LCDs (one for each beam) and being recomposed before projection through the lens system.

Another technology widely used for video projection is Digital Light Processing (DLP). In DLP projectors, the image is created by microscopically small mirrors laid out in a matrix on a semiconductor chip, known as a Digital Micromirror Devices (DMDs). Each mirror represents one or more pixels in the projected image, and the number of mirrors corresponds to the resolution of the projected image. These mirrors can be rapidly repositioned to reflect light either through the lens or onto a heat sink. Quickly toggling the mirror between these two orientations (essentially, on and off) produces grayscales, controlled by the ratio of on-time to off-time.

Depending on the light source, different methods exist to create color images with DLP projectors. With white lamps, a color wheel divided into multiple sectors (primary additive and subtractive colors) is placed between the lamp and the DLP and synchronized with the latter. The projector then displays consecutively images of each color of the wheel. A color breakup phenomenon, known as "rainbow effect", may then appear due to this succession of single-colored images. In most recent video projectors with multicolor LEDs or laser sources, no color wheel is needed, as color change can reach higher frequencies than with color wheels (up to 2000 Hz[20]). Similar to tri-LCD projectors, some video projectors use a tri-DLP system to get rid of the spinning color wheel. The light source is split into three primary colors before going to three DLP (one for each beam) and being recomposed before projection through the lens system.

#### 3.1.1.4  Stereoscopy

In Head-Mounted Displays (HMDs), the mechanical design allows each eye to only see a dedicated part of the screen or their dedicated screen for high-end versions. To render stereoscopy—namely, dedicated images for left and right eyes—in other visualization systems such as CAVEs or simulators, most of these installations use specific glasses. These stereoscopic glasses can either use passive or active filtering. Passive filtering constantly forwards the appropriate stream from the binocular input to each eye, whereas active filtering uses electronics to filter it and synchronize it with the display system.

With active filtering, images for the left and right eyes are displayed alternatively by the display system (see Fig. 3.2). The active stereoscopic glasses are equipped with liquid crystal active shutters blocking the image to the appropriate eye in synchronization with the incoming stream. The resulting image frequency for each eye is

---

[20]Norxe P1: https://www.norxe.com/p1/.

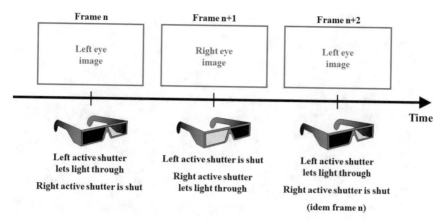

**Fig. 3.2** Active stereoscopy principle. Images for the left and right eyes are displayed alternatively by the display system. The active stereoscopic glasses are equipped with liquid crystal active shutters blocking the image to the appropriate eye in synchronization with the incoming stream

then halved from the incoming source. This method can be achieved with either video projectors or screens and makes it possible to keep the full color spectrum. However, the resulting perceived brightness gets decreased since the glasses shut the light out half of the time, and they are slightly dark even when they let the light through, as they are polarized. By increasing the image source frequency (frames per second), it is possible to have a multiuser experience, with projectors going up to 360 Hz and allowing three users to have a stereoscopic image on the same screen with a 60 Hz frequency image on each eye.[21] It is also possible to have a "pactive" (combination of passive and active) technology by adding active shutters in front of two standard video projectors and synchronize them with the glasses to achieve 60 Hz for each eye with two projectors displaying at 60 Hz. Fakespace proposed this technology (Machover and Encarnação 2006), but having two stages of shuttering in the light path decreases the perceived brightness even more and can add some latency due to synchronization issues between all the active shutters.

With passive filtering, stereoscopic glasses constantly filter incoming light according to wavelength or polarization, depending on the technology used. Based on wavelength, anaglyph is a well-known and low-cost method to encode each eye's image using two different complementary colors, typically red and cyan. In this method, no filter is required on the image source, only on the glasses, as the left and right images are "coded" in the image. The left eye will then see the red part of the image source, and the right eye the cyan part (green and blue). The anaglyph method can be used on any display system and requires only low-cost glasses. However, the main disadvantage is that the colors viewed will always be wrong since each eye is getting only part of the RGB color range. Users may also experience "ghosting" effects when some color from the left image gets into the right eye (or vice versa).

---

[21]Digital Projection INSIGHT 4 K HFR 360: https://www.digitalprojection.com/emea/dp-projectors/insight-4k-hfr-360.

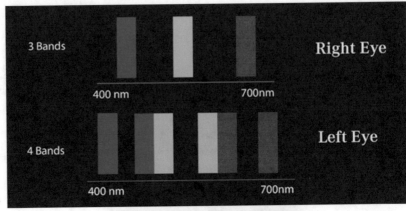

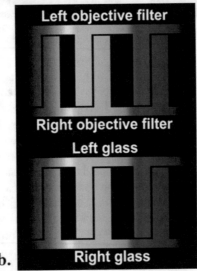

**Fig. 3.3** Examples of interference filter wavelength splitting for **a** Infitec and **b** Dolby 3D (https://commons.wikimedia.org/wiki/File:Dolby3d_Filters.png3dnatureguy/CCBY-SA)

A more recent passive stereoscopy method based on wavelength is interference filter systems (see Fig. 3.3). This technique uses specific wavelengths of red, green, and blue for the right eye, and different wavelengths of red, green, and blue for the left eye. Special interference filters (dichromatic filters) are used both in the glasses and in the projector to allow the wearer to see a color image with each eye. Different standards exist for interference filter systems: Infitec (a Daimler spin-off) and, proposed by most professional video projectors makers,[22] Dolby 3D and Panavision 3D (discontinued since 2012). Interference filter systems can only be used with video projectors and require at least two of them (one for the left eye image and

---

[22]Infitec: https://infitec.net/professional-solutions/.

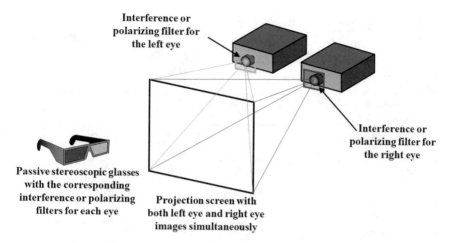

**Fig. 3.4** Illustration of passive stereoscopy filtering with interference filters or polarizing filters

one for the right eye image) because of the specific optical filter in each. In contrast, the anaglyph technique or active filtering can be used with a single video projector. The perceived brightness can then reach high values more easily than with active stereoscopy, as two video projectors are used instead of one, and each eye sees a continuous video stream (i.e., there is no alternation between left and right eyes).

Another widely used passive stereoscopy method is polarizing filters. To present stereoscopic images and films, two images are projected superimposed onto the same projection screen through different polarizing filters (see Fig. 3.4). The viewer wears low-cost eyeglasses that contain a pair of different polarizing filters. As each filter passes only the light which is similarly polarized and blocks the light polarized in the opposite direction, each eye sees a different image. Similar to interference filter systems, this method can be used only with video projectors and requires at least two of them. Furthermore, it involves the use of a specific projection screen (silver screen) to prevent the reflected light (or transmitted light for rear projection) seen by the user from losing its polarization. This method is widely used in theaters, as the cost and the weight of polarized glasses are very low compared to interference filter glasses or active shutter glasses.

In all the above-described display systems, a pair of eyeglasses is always necessary (see Table 3.2), which adds some discomfort to the user and reduces their field of view. To overcome this limitation, some display systems render stereoscopy without using glasses and are then called autostereoscopic display systems. Some of them also render the full light field—namely, the rendering of stereoscopy, accommodation, vergence, and motion parallax like in real conditions—and will be described below.

**Table 3.2** Comparison of main stereoscopy methods

|  | Active filtering (shutter glasses) | Anaglyph | Interference filtering | Polarizing filtering |
|---|---|---|---|---|
| Glasses requiring power | Yes | No | No | No |
| Glasses requiring synchronization | Yes | No | No | No |
| Weight of the glasses | High | Low | Low | Low |
| Price of the glasses | High | Low | High | Low |
| Compatible with screens | Yes | Yes | No | No |
| Compatible with video projectors | Yes | Yes | Yes | Yes |
| Minimum number of video projectors | 1 | 1 | 2 | 2 |
| Color spectrum loss | No | Yes | Yes | No |
| Brightness loss | Yes | No | No | Yes |
| Possibility of multiuser experience | Yes | No | No | No |

### 3.1.1.5  Autostereoscopic Display Systems

Autostereoscopy is mainly based on lenticular lenses or parallax barriers (Dodgson 2005; Järvenpää and Salmimaa 2008); see Fig. 3.5. The left and right images are cut into strips and then interlaced to form interwoven strips. The display renders a stereoscopic image either through a parallax barrier or a lenticular lens made of half-cylindrical lenses of the size of one interlaced left-right strip, and each interlaced

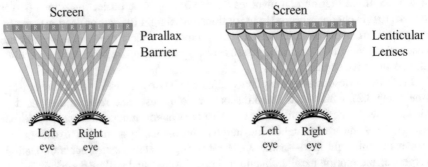

**a. Autostereoscopic display system with parallax barrier**

**b. Autostereoscopic display system with lenticular lenses**

**Fig. 3.5** Illustrations of autostereoscopic display systems with parallax barrier (**a**) or lenticular lenses (**b**)

strip is displayed through each lens. The human eyes perceive each strip accordingly, and the brain fuses the left and right strip to build an image including depth.

The main advantage of autostereoscopic displays is that they do not require users to wear glasses as in CAVEs. Some on-the-shelf products use them like, for instance, the range of screens sold by Alioscopy with a patented lenticular array.[23] The Nintendo 3DS game console uses a parallax barrier to allow for stereoscopic images without glasses. [24] Some reviews criticize the fact that this "3D" feature, in addition to halving resolution by two, forced the user to maintain the game console at a constant distance and orientation so that the stereoscopy works.[25] Although Nintendo 3DS sales were at a comparable level from other portable consoles of Nintendo, the "3D feature" has not been reconducted to next generation consoles.

More generally, many autostereoscopic displays are single-view displays and are thus not capable of reproducing the sense of movement parallax. Some autostereo-scopic displays, however, are multi-view displays and render one image per viewpoint thanks to multiple video projectors, as proposed, for example, by Holografika. This feature can be used in collaborative applications but only allows left-right movement parallax and not top-down.

The major drawbacks of such technology are the following: (i) lenticular lenses require high precision manufacturing to enable accurate image rendering; (ii) pixel density is limited by the size of the lenticular lens; (iii) display resolution is divided by the number of viewpoints in case of multiple viewpoints; (iv) luminance may not be distributed uniformly (Salmimaa and Järvenpää 2008; Pölönen et al. 2011); (v) in the case of multiple viewpoints, space is needed for video projectors, unless small-sized video projectors with low image resolutions are used; (vi) in case of multiple viewpoints, motion parallax can be reproduced only in one direction (usually, left-right), which does not take user's height into account.

### 3.1.1.6 Light Field Rendering

Autostereoscopic displays rendering the full light field were developed to overcome the abovementioned limitations deriving from autostereoscopic displays using lenticular lenses or a parallax barrier. In the middle of the twentieth century, Gershun (1939) formalized the concept of light field by describing the luminosity of a given point as a function of both its position and the directions of all rays coming from all light sources (active or passive). It is only at the end of the century that Adelson and Bergen (1991) defined the plenoptic function as an application of light field analysis for computational graphics imaging. The function has five parameters and delivers the luminance of a certain point $x, y, z$ seen under a direction defined by two angles $\theta$ and $\phi$, thus providing a complete holographic representation of a visual environment

---

[23] Alioscopy Glasses-Free 3D Displays: http://www.alioscopy.com/en/3Ddisplays.php.

[24] Nintendo 3DS: https://en.wikipedia.org/wiki/Nintendo_3DS.

[25] Engadget, Nintendo 3DS review, 2011: https://www.engadget.com/2011-03-21-nintendo-3ds-review.html.

(Fig. 3.6). This function could also be extrapolated to two additional parameters: time $t$ and light's wavelength $\lambda$.

This idealized function has been simplified to four dimensions by Levoy and Hanrahan (1996) with a pair of points in two arbitrary planes (see Fig. 3.7). This 4D light field representation has allowed using traditional pictures to recreate the plenoptic function. The key to this technique lies in interpreting the input images as 2D slices of the 4D function—the light field. This function fully characterizes the flow of light through unobstructed space in a static scene with fixed illumination.

Several techniques exist to render this light field, the most well-known being holography. Another technique, suggested by Lanman et al. (2010), Wetzstein et al. (2011), consists of using multiple LCD screens in multiple layers (two layers for Lanman and five for Wetzstein) in order to combine them in a multiplicative manner.

**Fig. 3.6** Representation of the 5D plenoptic function giving the luminance L as a function of the coordinates (x, y, z) of the considered point and the viewing direction defined by the angles $\theta$ and $\phi$

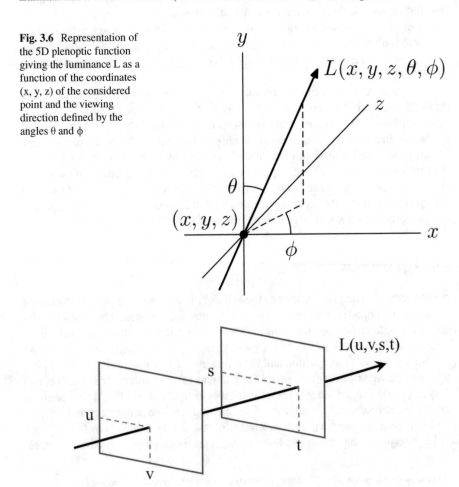

**Fig. 3.7** Graphic representation of a parameterization of a 4D light field, as proposed by Levoy and Hanrahan (1996)

This technique shows to be brighter and with higher resolution than techniques of lenslet array or parallax barrier with a similar form factor. The "light field stereoscope" proposed by Huang et al. (2015) is the first wearable display using a two-layer LCD setup to display a 4D light field to each eye. The user is then provided with stereoscopic cues (binocular disparity) as well as monoscopic focus cues with the light field. More recently, a prototype called "Aktina Vision" was made able to reproduce over 100 million light rays at angle intervals of less than 1° with a maximum resolution of approximately 330,000 pixels (Watanabe et al. 2019). Despite the interesting potential of light field technology, off-the-shelf commercial systems have not yet been proposed, though Holografika's Holovision (Balogh and Kovács 2010), dedicated mostly to research and special events, is commercially available.

### 3.1.2 A Brief History of HMDs

We mentioned in Chap. 1 that the first VR Head-Mounted Display (HMD) was introduced by Sutherland in 1968. However, the idea of a pair of goggles that display imaginary worlds is older. The American writer Stanley G. Weinbaum wrote in 1935 a short story, *Pygmalion's Spectacles*, featuring a professor who invented a pair of goggles enabling "a movie that gives one sight and sound […] taste, smell, and touch. […] You are in the story, you speak to the shadows (characters) and they reply, and instead of being on a screen, the story is all about you, and you are in it" (Weinbaum 1935).

Twenty-five years passed before the very first head-mounted display was patented by Morton Heilig[26] and called it the Telesphere Mask (Heilig 1960). This HMD enabled stereoscopy and stereo-sound but no motion tracking. In 1961, the Headsight HMD was invented to project distant images with head motion tracking embedded. However, this HMD was not aimed at VR applications yet.

Then came the already-mentioned Sutherland's Sword of Damocles in 1968, which enabled projecting wire-framed images.

In 1986, Tom Furness presented the Super Cockpit developed for the pilots of the US Air Force, consisting of a helmet that could project computer-generated information, imagery from radars, and data into a real-time virtual space (Furness 1986). The HMD was embedded with a tracking system, voice controls, and sensors allowing controlling the aircraft with gestures, voice, and eye movements.

In parallel, the commercialization of VR HMD started in 1985 by VPL under the name EyePhone. A collaboration between VPL and the NASA led to the development in the late 1980s of the Virtual Interface Environment Workstation (VIEW) composed of an HMD with LCD displays that could display computer-generated images and a

---

[26]Morton Heilig (1926–1997) was a cinematrographer. He is known to have invented the Sensorama in 1957, a machine for viewing movies with full sensory immersion (stereoscopy, motion, fans, odor, stereo-sound) (Heilig 1962), and which is considered as the very first VR system.

head position tracking system. A data glove and a data suit complemented the system for full interaction with the content (Fisher et al. 1987, 1988).

The 1990s witnessed the development of HMDs for video games, such as Sega's VR headset, VictorMaxx's CyberMaxx, or Nintendo's Virtual Boy. However, most of them were either not released (e.g., the Sega VR) or a commercial failure occurred (e.g., Nintendo's Virtual Boy). Indeed, as for the Virtual Boy, the HMD was heavy, displayed only red and black images which was uncomfortable, and had a low resolution.

Despite these fails, the industry quickly found interest in virtual reality technologies for product development. Several HMDs were released in the 1990s and the 2000s for professionals and used, for instance, by the driving simulation community. Among them, we can cite the n-Vision that was used at Volvo (Burns and Saluäär 1999), the Kaiser Electro-Optics ProView VL50 and SEOS HMDs that were adopted at Renault (Coates et al. 2002; Fuchs 2017), and the Sensics XSight HMD used at Volkswagen with a robot-based cybermotion simulator (Grabe et al. 2010). Compared to early HMDs dedicated to video games, these HMDs were high-class products, with already advanced characteristics, such as $1,920 \times 1,200$ pixels per eye and a $123°$ field of view for the Sensics XSight, which, looking at today's HMDs, was impressive. However, they were expensive and could be heavy.

The years 2010 marked the beginning of the era of affordable virtual reality helmets as we know them today. In 2010, Palmer Luckey—an 18-year-old entrepreneur—created the first prototype of the Oculus Rift with a $90°$ field of view, but the first commercialized version was released in 2012 after a successful Kickstarter campaign that raised US$2.4 million. In 2014, Oculus was bought by Facebook for US$2 billion. Since then, many big companies have developed their own HMD to be commercialized at affordable prices. The list includes Sony PlayStation VR, Google Cardboard, Samsung Gear VR (which was actually developed with Oculus), HTC Vive, and Microsoft WMR. Furthermore, dozens of startups emerged and competed with each other to provide the best VR HMD.

In 2015, Microsoft presented the HoloLens, which gained keen interest among end users, especially in the industrial field. However, the field of view is low (around $35°$), and the helmet cannot be worn for a long time due to its weight. The HoloLens 2 was then released in 2019 with around twice the field of view of the first version.

Also to be mentioned are the Magic Leap One glasses, released in 2018, which are claimed to use light field technologies.

## 3.2  Sensory Excitation Through Motion Platform

### 3.2.1  Type of Motion Systems and Motion Technologies

#### 3.2.1.1  Hexapods and Other Parallel Robots

Many different mechanical architectures are used in simulations; however, we can notice the generalization of parallel platforms. Parallel robots have the advantage of providing accurate positioning because the measurement and positioning errors at the individual joints are averaged, whereas they are cumulated on a serial robot. In addition, parallel robots can move a larger load than serial robots. In a parallel robot, the load is distributed over the individual actuators, whereas in a serial robot, each actuator must support the entire load. This aspect is crucial, as the moving mass of driving or flight simulators (which includes the cockpit, the screen, the video projectors, the air conditioning, etc.) can reach many tons. In the 1970s, Gough and Stewart proposed a parallel robot architecture with 6 degrees of freedom (DOF), which is widely used in simulation (flight or driving). Their robot is composed of two approximately triangular-shaped plates and six cylinders connecting the vertices of the triangles.

Cylinders can be either hydraulic, pneumatic, or electric. In the first two cases, they are "piston" actuators whose valves (usually servo valves) control the flow of oil or air at the inlet. The flow rate is regulated according to the difference between the current and the desired elongations of the cylinder. Electric cylinders are ball screw-nut systems. An electric motor rotates the nut part of the cylinder, which causes the rod (the screw part of the cylinder) to extend. The piloting is then carried out by controlling the rotation of the motor.

Electric jacks have the advantage of being less expensive and easier to maintain. However, hydraulic or pneumatic cylinders can develop more power and can reach higher linear speeds and frequencies (electric cylinders usually being not able to render frequencies above 50 Hz). One of their disadvantages, however, is that they require a power unit (hydraulic or pneumatic) to pressurize the oil or air supplied to the cylinders.

#### 3.2.1.2  Rails

Acceleration restitution is usually achieved through a combination of two techniques. The first part of the accelerations (the high-frequency part) is directly rendered by the movements of the motion system. Another part (the low-frequency part) is rendered by tilt coordination (see below, 3.2.2). The main drawback of this way of proceeding is that it is difficult to obtain full complementarity of these two techniques, as the tilt coordination only allows rendering accelerations at low frequency. Specifically, what is not reproduced by one of the two techniques is not necessarily reproduced by the other. Furthermore, some parts of the motion to render could be missing.

It was not possible to indefinitely increase the size of the parallel robots, in the context of driving simulations where horizontal accelerations can be higher both in terms of amplitude and frequency than in flight simulations. Hence, motion systems with rails were developed to increase the duration of motion cues on the horizontal level. These simulators with an 8-DOF architecture always use a Gough–Stewart platform whose base, instead of being fixed to the ground, is mounted on a double rail structure (XY rails) allowing horizontal deflections of several meters. The first simulator using this architecture was the University of Iowa's National Advanced Driving Simulator (NADS), which was started in 1992 and became operational in 2002 (see Fig. 3.8). It has a horizontal deflection of 20 m, both longitudinally and laterally (Greenberg et al. 2006).

This simulator has been followed by many others, such as Renault's ULTIMATE simulator, allowing 6 × 6 m of horizontal displacements (Dagdelen et al. 2006), Toyota's driving simulator in Japan, VTI's driving simulators in Sweden, or Daimler driving simulator in Germany (Fig. 3.9).

Most recent driving simulator motion systems integrate a yaw table allowing to turn the cabin around the yaw axis. As for the addition of rails to the hexapod, this turntable addition comes from a specific need of driving simulation compared to flight simulation, as this kind of motion is needed for the reproduction of 90° turns or roundabouts, among others.

Since the first driving simulators using X-Y rails, the technology has remarkably improved. Most recent rail motion systems in driving simulators use linear motor

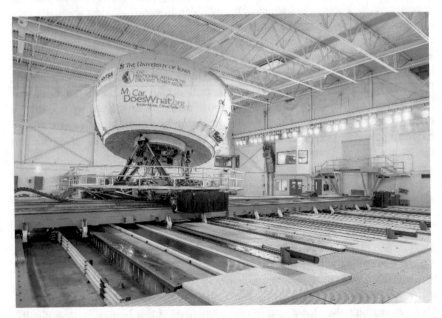

**Fig. 3.8** University of Iowa's National Advanced Driving Simulator (NADS) Greenberg et al. (2006)

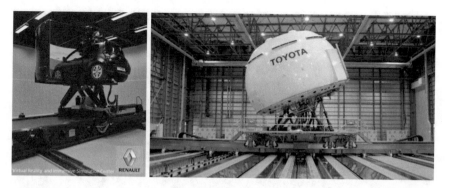

**Fig. 3.9** Dynamic driving simulators from Renault (ULTIMATE) and Toyota

technology, the first one being Daimler's Moving Base Simulator MBS2 (Klüver et al. 2015), followed by Nissan's driving simulator, the future dynamic driving simulators of Renault (Bosch Rexroth 2018a) and BMW (Bosch Rexroth 2018b), among others. Linear motors use the same principle than standard electric motors, namely, the attraction-repulsion forces generated between a current-carrying coil and a magnet. In the case of linear motors, the permanent magnets are disposed horizontally, and the moving part contains coils supplied with power depending on the desired acceleration or force. The main advantages of this kind of solution are its lower latency and higher smoothness (when changing direction) than standard "rack and pinion" solutions. However, its price is generally higher, and its installation is more complicated due to the small and constant air gap that needs to be maintained between the coils (moving part) and the permanent magnets (static part) for the optimal performance of the linear motors.

### 3.2.1.3 Other Motion Systems

Gough–Stewart platforms and rails are the most common parts of simulators' motion systems, yet not the only ones. A large variety of other technical solutions exist, some of which are presented here.

The VI-grade company launched the Driver in Motion (DiM) range of driving simulators in which the rails and the yaw table are replaced by three horizontal actuators that make it possible to translate and rotate the base of the hexapod in the horizontal direction, the latter being on an air cushion (see Fig. 3.10). This technical solution is limited in terms of displacements (up to 2.5 m); nonetheless, it delivers higher stiffness and bandwidth.

Both the Max Planck Institute for Biological Cybernetics in Tübingen and the German Aerospace Center (DLR) have developed a simulator based on a robotic arm mounted on a rail (see Fig. 3.11). The TNO in the Netherlands, for its part, has developed a simulator called Desdemona with centrifugal architecture, which

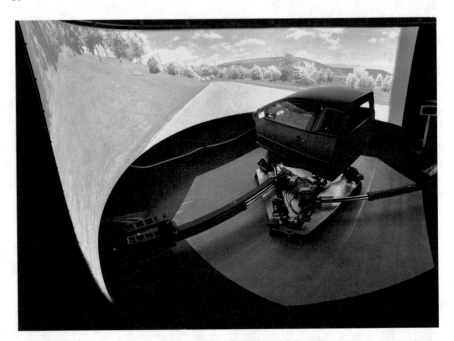

**Fig. 3.10**  VI-grade's DiM platform (Bruschetta et al. 2018)

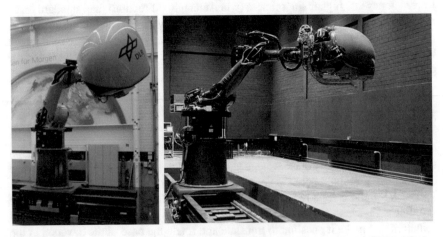

**Fig. 3.11**  Simulators based on a robotic arm from the German Aerospace Center (DLR) (Fischer et al. 2015) and the Max Planck Institute for Biological Cybernetics (Venrooij et al. 2015)

provides unlimited rendering accelerations yet requires complex algorithms for its motion cueing due to its unique architecture (see Fig. 3.12).

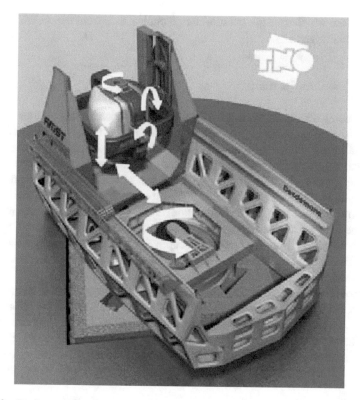

**Fig. 3.12** Desdemona Simulator from TNO, based on a centrifugal architecture (Wentink et al. 2008)

## 3.2.2 Motion Cueing

The transformation from a vehicle's (i.e., an automobile, an aircraft, and a train) dynamics to simulator displacements is called motion cueing. The main function of the motion cueing algorithm (MCA) is to reproduce a motion perception for the driver or pilot as close as possible to what the latter would have perceived in real conditions. As the motion capabilities of a motion system are by nature more restrictive than those of a real vehicle, the MCA must keep the simulator's motion system within its physical limits, for all its degrees of freedom, in excursions as well as in velocities and accelerations. As achieving the highest motion rendering fidelity generally implies having significant displacements, carrying out these functions often leads to contradictory constraints.

To fulfill these two objectives, MCAs use different approaches, from simple filtering in the "classical" MCA to Model Predictive Control (MPC) in recent developments. MCA also uses knowledge from human motion perception, such as perception thresholds and perception ambiguities. The most well-known technique is tilt coordination, which uses the gravito-inertial equivalence from the otolith organs in the vestibular system.

### 3.2.2.1 Tilt Coordination

Motion cueing often uses the technique known as tilt coordination (Nahon and Reid 1990), which takes advantage of the sensory ambiguity of the otolith organs between horizontal accelerations and gravity inclination (see Chap. 2, Sect. 2.1.2) to reproduce the sensations of sustained accelerations in the horizontal plane. The tilt coordination technique consists of tilting the user so that a part of the gravity is interpreted as a longitudinal acceleration (see Fig. 3.13). The tilt of the driver stimulates their otoliths in the same way as a horizontal acceleration, thus causing the illusion. For example, tilting the user backward will provoke the illusion of being accelerated forward. Tilting the user also stimulates the proprioceptive system, namely, the pressure forces of the seat or the seat belt and the perceived effects of the entire motion system, which either complements or modifies the perceived vestibular cues.

To provide a coherent perception of horizontal accelerations, the other sensory cues—in particular, visual cues—must be adequately generated. Therefore, if the display system is not attached to the platform or cabin, the image must be corrected so that the visual environment remains stable for the driver. Furthermore, the tilting must be performed at a speed below the detection threshold of the semicircular channels—3°/s according to Groen and Bles (2004), 5°/s for roll tilt rendering in

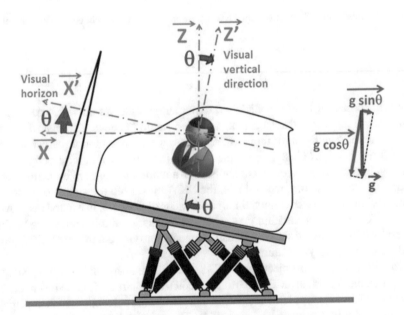

**Fig. 3.13** Illustration of the tilt coordination technique (Colombet et al. 2015)

driving simulations (Fang et al. 2014), and 6°/s for pitch tilt rendering (Colombet et al. 2015).

It is generally admitted that the rotation of the driver for tilt coordination should be realized around a point located in the middle of their two vestibular systems. According to Reymond and Kemeny (2000), it could be located even above the head for a better rendering of proprioceptive stimuli (i.e., with seat pressure on the back). Tilt coordination rotations are never exactly around the head's center as it would require tracking the latter in real time during the simulation, besides considering it as MCA input. The undesired linear accelerations induced by decentering are then generally neglected, as they often are below the perception threshold or neglectable when compared to other vehicle linear accelerations.

### 3.2.2.2 Classical Filtering

Initially developed by Schmidt and Conrad (1970) for flight simulators, the classical motion cueing algorithm is the most widely used algorithm in commercial simulators. The vehicle linear and angular accelerations are high-pass filtered using second-order filters to maintain the motion system in its workspace (Fig. 3.14). A third-order filter is applied to return (or washout) the motion base to its neutral position (Reid and Nahon 1985). An "anti-backlash" filter is added by Reymond and Kemeny (2000) in their implementation to reduce certain artifacts that are induced by the high-pass filters. The vehicle longitudinal and lateral accelerations are low-pass filtered, scaled, and passed through rate limiters to produce additional pitch and roll "tilt coordination" angles. The parameters of the classical MCA must be tuned to guarantee that the outputs are always consistent with the platform limits, which is generally done by considering a "worst-case" driving situation in terms of acceleration amplitude and duration. Therefore, in normal driving conditions, only part of the platform capacities are used (Figs. 3.13 and 3.14).

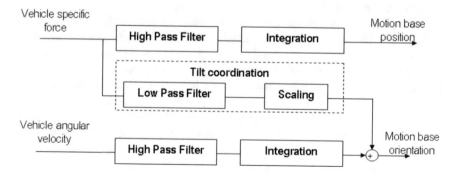

**Fig. 3.14** Classical Motion Cueing Algorithm filter structure (Colombet et al. 2008)

### 3.2.2.3  Adaptive Filtering

In an attempt to improve the classical strategy—in particular, the adjustment of parameters—Parrish et al. (1975) proposed the so-called adaptive strategy, which was later developed by Reid and Nahon (1985). Its structure is based on that of the classical approach. The difference lies in the parameters ($\alpha$) of the filters, which are no longer constant during the simulation. They are recalculated at each time step to minimize a cost function $J(\alpha)$ defined as

$$J(\alpha) = [\text{Acc}_{\text{veh}} - \text{Acc}_{\text{MS}}]^2 + \omega_1 [\text{Vel}_{\text{MS}}]^2 + \omega_2 [\text{Pos}_{\text{MS}}]^2$$

The first term corresponds to the difference between the acceleration of the simulated vehicle and the acceleration of the motion system calculated by the algorithm. The other two terms involving the velocity and the position of the motion system are used to limit the movements of the platform and return it to its neutral position. The two weighting factors $\omega_1$ and $\omega_2$ allow the user to adjust the compromise between the fidelity of the restitution and the respect of the physical limits.

The result is a nonlinear strategy that, compared to the classical strategy, increases the fidelity of the restitution of accelerations around the neutral position. However, there are always parameters to be set ($\omega_1$ and $\omega_2$)—a task that is always performed by trial and error and is not obvious to inexperienced users. Furthermore, the user will not be sure that the physical limits are not exceeded.

### 3.2.2.4  Model Predictive Control

To overcome the problems raised by the previous MCA, Dagdelen (2005) proposes a new approach based on the Model-based Predictive Control (MPC) technique. This MPC MCA explicitly takes (i) a human motion perception model, (ii) the physical constraints of the simulator's motion system, and (iii) a dynamic model of the platform into account.

This nonlinear approach calculates the trajectory set point to be provided to the platform at each time step to both minimize the perceived acceleration deviation using a human perception model and keep the simulator within its position, speed, and acceleration limits by explicitly using its physical constraints over a specific time horizon. Furthermore, the calculated trajectory is applied only if the simulator can be stopped with an imperceptible deceleration (i.e., below the perception threshold) before reaching the position limits. Moreover, a specific part of the algorithm must be implemented to return (or washout) the platform to neutral when it reaches a limit position.

This approach, by explicitly considering a perceptual model and the simulator's physical limits, ensures better use of the workspace while minimizing sensory conflicts. In addition, the user, this time, is assured not to send an order exceeding the physical limits. These results have been tested and validated for the first time on the

Renault ULTIMATE simulator (Dagdelen et al. 2004). Since then, a lot of comparative studies have been carried out in driving simulation and the MPC MCA seems to have obtained a consensus from both the scientific community and the driving simulator users. The works from Venrooij et al. (2016) and Lamprecht et al. (2019) on the Daimler driving simulator indicate a clear subjective preference in passive drivers for MPC MCA compared to filter-based MCA. The continuous work of Fang during the last years (Fang et al. 2018, 2019) may enhance the prediction of the algorithm and thus increase its performance, namely, its ability to reduce the acceleration perception difference between the real vehicle and the simulator. Finally, with the MPC-MCA variant from Bruschetta et al. (2018), a novel cost function was proposed to enhance drivers' perception of their vehicle in the context of race circuits.

## 3.3 Walking Systems

To prevent the sensory conflict described in Sect. 2.3.1 from occurring while traveling in immersive environments, real walking represents the best travel modality. However, limited physical traveling space constraints impose to find alternatives. In Chap. 4, we present several computer-based means to alleviate cybersickness effects. Another way to address the sensory conflict issue is to enable users to physically move as close to reality as possible, thanks to hardware setups.

### 3.3.1 Unidirectional Treadmills

Diverted from its primary use in sports training, the unidirectional treadmill is probably the first device one can think of to try to reproduce a natural walk. The user's position along the treadmill is measured to keep the latter centered by adjusting its running speed. This device has many limitations, which are common to most locomotion interfaces. The surface of the belt is smooth and uniform and cannot reflect the range of textures that a virtual floor could have (e.g., asphalt, carpet, and sand). Since the surface is flat, no relief can be transcribed (e.g., slope, descent, and stairs). Similarly, nothing prevents the user from entering a wall and it allows them to move in only one direction. A rotation control is then necessary if one wishes to have more degrees of freedom. Several variants try to overcome these problems.

The *Sarcos Treadport* (Hollerbach et al. 2000) is composed of a conveyor belt mounted on a single-axis rotating platform and a motorized mechanical harness allowing the transfer of forces on three axes. This device makes it possible to simulate slopes by playing on the inclination and prevent the user from walking in the walls by blocking the scrolling of the belt and the harness.

The *ATR Locomotion Interface for Active Self Motion* (ATR ATLAS) (Noma 1998) consists of an active treadmill mounted on a three-axis rotating platform. By acting on roll and pitch, it can simulate slopes in all directions. The yaw is used to allow the user to change direction. An optical tracking system retrieves the positions of the user's feet, whose movement is then analyzed to anticipate and cancel direction changes and stabilize the user in the center of the mat. An improved version—the *ATR Ground Surface Simulator* (GSS) (Noma et al. 2000)—makes it possible to re-transcribe the relief of the terrain in a richer way than the solutions playing on the slope of the mat. Here, electric jacks present under the surface of the treadmill dynamically modify its profile to simulate slopes of more complex shapes.

### 3.3.2 Omnidirectional Treadmills

Several prototypes of omnidirectional treadmills have been developed to allow the user to move infinitely in two directions in space. There are two main variants.

The *roller belt* (Darken et al. 1997) is made up of two treadmills assembled perpendicularly. As for a conventional unidirectional treadmill, the outer belt can cancel the user's movements in one direction. For the perpendicular direction, the inner belt drives small free rollers located in the outer belt. A harness mechanically measures the users' position and the users are constantly redirected toward the center of the device so that they never reach the edge of the device, which can only be used by one user at a time.

The *toroidal treadmill* (Iwata 1999) is the successor of the roller conveyor, and it consists of a multitude of treadmills linked together to form a macro treadmill. The combined surface of the belts forms a torus—hence the name. The system can reach large dimensions, as is the case with the *CyberWalk* (Souman et al. 2008), and it can compensate for the user's movements without any noticeable acceleration of the belt. Furthermore, the user can walk, accelerate, change direction, and suddenly stop without ever reaching the edge of the mat. The toroidal treadmill is the ultimate device to explore large spaces in an immersive way. However, in combination with a VR helmet, issues of confidence in the system arise: the user is so free that he may be afraid to reach the edge of the mat.

### 3.3.3 Gait Devices

The peculiarity of this device is that each foot is treated individually. In the case of the *GAIT system* (Iwata et al. 2001), two motorized plates, each with two axes of translation, act as a virtual floor by being placed at each moment where the user is likely to put his foot. The whole thing is mounted on a rotating platform that accompanies the user's rotational movements. The device makes it possible to simulate the ascent or descent of stairs by controlling the elevation of the plates, which allows movements on three axes. The device remains constraining, however, because the user must always hold on to a bar and can only perform movements of small amplitude. The *Sarcos Biport* (Hollerbach 2002) is based on haptics since the user's feet are linked to force feedback arms, which allows movements with six degrees of freedom. The system constantly returns the user to his initial position and orientation.

### 3.3.4  Walking Spheres

This device works on a principle similar to that of a ball mouse. It consists of a sphere in which the user can walk or run in any direction. This sphere can be supported by bearings or on an air cushion, and its peculiarity is its passivity: thanks to the spherical geometry of the device, the centering of the users is produced by their walking. The diameter of the sphere is crucial because a large sphere makes it possible to feel the curvature of the ground less, thus improving the immersion. A head-mounted display can be used to give a visual feedback, as is the case with the *Virtusphere* (Medina et al. 2008), or the image can be projected back onto the surface of the device, as with the *Cybersphere* (Fernandes et al. 2003).

### 3.3.5  Ball Carpets

The *Omnidirectional Ball-Bearing Disc Platform* (OBDP) (Huang et al. 2000) is a spherical ball mat composed of a portion of a sphere lined with spring-loaded balls. The user is held in its center by a physical structure surrounding the platform and walks on the mat. The spherical shape allows the user to be brought back to the center at all times, which makes it a passive device. The depression of each ball is measured to detect footprints. A computer vision algorithm calculates the balls' movements to estimate the user's movements.

The *CyberCarpet* (De Luca et al. 2006) is an active device. It consists of a matrix of metal balls moved by a conveyor belt on a rotating platform. The device is small and does not allow large displacements. Moreover, the prototype becomes unstable as soon as speed exceeds 1.5 m/s.

### 3.3.6  Walking Shoes

*Powered Shoes* (Iwata et al. 2006) operate on the inverse principle of motorized roller skates. Equipped with motorized wheels, they permanently compensate the user's movements, and their peculiarity is that they are portable. Nevertheless, the wheels of the shoes follow the foot's direction; hence, side steps cannot be compensated for.

The *String Walker* (Iwata et al. 2007) is based on the tension of strings. Each shoe has a smooth sole, attached by four wires to motorized systems, which are themselves connected to a rotating toric structure. The device allows movements in two axes and also manages side steps.

### 3.3.7  Mobile Tiles

Mobile tile systems such as *CirculaFloor* (Iwata et al. 2005) are composed of a network of robots that move independently yet coordinate to always be where the users put their foot. Some versions of the robots include a lifting platform to simulate virtual stair climbing. However, the prototype is still slow, hence not usable in practice.

### 3.3.8  Conclusion

Many walking systems have been proposed in the literature in the last 25 years to provide users with natural walking while being immersed in virtual environments. However, most of them were limited to research prototypes and were never commercialized.

In the last 5 years, several companies attempted to offer on-the-shelf walking systems, mostly for the entertainment market. Among them are the *Virtuix Omni,*[27] the *Cyberith Virtualizer,*[28] the *KAT Walk,*[29] and the *Infinadeck,*[30] available in the market. Most of these systems rely on a low friction surface with sometimes special shoes to be used, allowing users to walk as naturally as possible. However, these systems require users to be harnessed to prevent them from falling, which can be constraining.

### References

Adelson EH, Bergen JR (1991) The plenoptic function and the elements of early vision. Computational models of visual processing. MIT Press, Cambridge, MA, pp 3–20

Balogh T, Kovács PT (2010) Real-time 3D light field transmission. In: Real-time image and video processing 2010. International Society for Optics and Photonics, p 772406

Bosch Rexroth (2018a) Bosch Rexroth delivers advanced motion platform for Renault simulator I Bosch Rexroth AG. https://www.boschrexroth.com/en/xc/company/press/index2-31040. Accessed 10 Apr 2020

---

[27] Virtuix: https://www.virtuix.com/.

[28] Cyberith: https://www.cyberith.com/.

[29] Kat VR: https://www.kat-vr.com/.

[30] Infinadek: https://infinadeck.com/.

Bosch Rexroth (2018b) High-fidelity and high-dynamic driving simulators for testing autonomous driving solutions and vehicle dynamics | Bosch Rexroth AG. https://www.boschrexroth.com/en/xc/company/press/index2-32832. Accessed 10 Apr 2020

Bruschetta M, Mendola DL, Beghi A, Minen D (2018) An MPC based Motion Cueing Algorithm with side slip dynamics. In: Proceedings of the driving simulation conference Europe. Antibes, France

Burns PC, Saluäär D (1999) Intersections between driving in reality and virtual reality (VR). pp 153–164

Coates N, Ehrette M, Hayes T, Blackham G, Heidet A, Kemeny A (2002) Head-mounted display in driving simulation applications in CARDS. In: Proceedings of the driving simulation conference

Colombet F, Dagdelen M, Reymond G, Pere C, Merienne F, Kemeny A (2008) Motion Cueing: what is the impact on the driver's behavior? In: Proceedings of the driving simulation conference Europe. Monaco, pp 171–181

Colombet F, Fang Z, Kemeny A (2015) Pitch tilt rendering for an 8-DOF driving simulator. Driving simulation conference 2015 Europe VR. DSC, Tübingen, Germany, pp 55–61

Dagdelen M (2005) Restitution des stimuli inertiels en simulation de conduite. Thesis, Paris, ENMP

Dagdelen M, Berlioux J-C, Panerai F, Reymond G, Kemeny A (2006) Validation process of the ULTIMATE high-performance driving simulator. In: Proceedings of the driving simulation conference. Paris, France, pp 37–48

Dagdelen M, Reymond G, Kemeny A, Bordier M, Maïzi N (2004) MPC based Motion Cueing Algorithm: development and application to the ULTIMATE driving simulator. In: Proceedings of the driving simulation conference Europe. Paris, France, pp 221–233

Darken RP, Cockayne WR, Carmein D (1997) The omni-directional treadmill: a locomotion device for virtual worlds. In: Proceedings of the 10th annual ACM symposium on User interface software and technology. Association for Computing Machinery, Banff, Alberta, Canada, pp 213–221

De Luca A, Mattone R, Giordano PR (2006) The motion control problem for the CyberCarpet. In: Proceedings 2006 IEEE international conference on robotics and Automation, 2006. ICRA 2006. pp 3532–3537

Dodgson NA (2005) Autostereoscopic 3D displays. Computer 38:31–36. https://doi.org/10.1109/MC.2005.252

Dolgoff E (1991) Active matrix LCD image projection system

Fang Z, Colombet F, Collinet J-C, Kemeny A (2014) Roll tilt thresholds for 8 DOF driving simulators. In: Proceedings of the driving simulation conference 2014 Europe. Paris, France

Fang Z, Tsushima M, Machida N, Colombet F, Wautier D, Kemeny A (2018) Fast MPC based MCA investigation and application. In: Proceedings of the driving simulation conference Europe. Antibes, France, pp 191–192

Fang Z, Wautier D, Kemeny A (2019) Development and applications of a fast MPC based motion cueing algorithm. In: Proceedings of the driving simulation conference Europe. Strasbourg, France, pp 109–116

Fernandes KJ, Raja V, Eyre J (2003) Cybersphere: the fully immersive spherical projection system. Commun ACM 46:141–146. https://doi.org/10.1145/903893.903929

Fischer M, Labusch A, Bellmann T, Seehof C (2015) A task-oriented catalogue of criteria for driving simulator evaluation. In: Proceedings of the driving simulation conference Europe. Tuebingen, Germany, pp 139–150

Fisher SS, McGreevy M, Humphries J, Robinett W (1987) Virtual environment display system. In: Proceedings of the 1986 workshop on Interactive 3D graphics. Association for Computing Machinery, Chapel Hill, North Carolina, USA, pp 77–87

Fisher SS, Wenzel EM, Coler C, McGreevy MW (1988) Virtual interface environment workstations. Proc Hum Factors Soc Annu Meet 32:91–95. https://doi.org/10.1177/154193128803200219

Fuchs P (2017) Virtual reality headsets—a theoretical and pragmatic approach. CRC Press

Furness TA (1986) The super cockpit and its human factors challenges. Proc Hum Factors Soc Annu Meet 30:48–52. https://doi.org/10.1177/154193128603000112

Gershun A (1939) The light field. J Math Phys 18:51–151. https://doi.org/10.1002/sapm193918151

Grabe V, Pretto P, Giordan PR, Bülthoff HH (2010) Influence of display type on drivers' performance in a motion-based driving simulator. In: Proceedings of the driving simulation conference 2010 Europe, pp 81–88

Greenberg J, Curry R, Blommer M, Kozak K, Artz B, Cathey L, Kao B (2006) The validity of last-second braking and steering judgements in advanced driving simulators. In: Proceedings of the driving simulation conference. Paris, France, pp 143–153

Groen EL, Bles W (2004) How to use body tilt for the simulation of linear self motion. J Vestib Res 14:375–385

Heilig ML (1962) Sensorama simulator

Heilig ML (1960) Stereoscopic-television apparatus for individual use

Hollerbach JM (2002) Locomotion interfaces. In: Handbook of virtual environments technology. Lawrence Erlbaum Associates, Inc., pp 239–254

Hollerbach JM, Xu Y, Christensen RR, Jacobsen SC (2000) Design specifications for the second generation Sarcos Treadport locomotion interface. In: Haptics symposium, asme dynamic systems and control division, DSC, pp 1293–1298

Huang F-C, Chen K, Wetzstein G (2015) The light field stereoscope: immersive computer graphics via factored near-eye light field displays with focus cues. ACM Trans Graph 34:60:1–60:12. https://doi.org/10.1145/2766922

Huang J, Chiu W, Lin Y, Tsai M, Bai H, Tai C, Gau C, Lee H (2000) The gait sensing disc—a compact locomotion device for the virtual environment. J WSCG

Iwata H (1999) The Torus Treadmill: realizing locomotion in VEs. IEEE Comput Grap Appl 19:30–35. https://doi.org/10.1109/38.799737

Iwata H, Yano H, Fukushima H, Noma H (2005) CirculaFloor [locomotion interface]. IEEE Comput Graph Appl 25:64–67. https://doi.org/10.1109/MCG.2005.5

Iwata H, Yano H, Nakaizumi F (2001) Gait Master: a versatile locomotion interface for uneven virtual terrain. Proc IEEE Virtual Reality 2001:131–137

Iwata H, Yano H, Tomioka H (2006) Powered shoes. In: ACM SIGGRAPH 2006 emerging technologies. Association for Computing Machinery, Boston, Massachusetts, pp 28–es

Iwata H, Yano H, Tomiyoshi M (2007) String walker. In: ACM SIGGRAPH 2007 emerging technologies. Association for Computing Machinery, San Diego, California, pp 20–es

Järvenpää T, Salmimaa M (2008) Optical characterization of autostereoscopic 3-D displays. J Soc Inform Display 16:825–833. https://doi.org/10.1889/1.2966444

Klüver M, Herrigel C, Preuß S, Schöner H-P, Hecht H (2015) Comparing the incidence of simulator sickness in five different driving simulators. In: Proceedings of the driving simulation conference. Tuebingen, Germany, pp 87–94

Lamprecht A, Steffen D, Haecker J, Graichen K (2019) Comparison between a Filter- and an MPC-based MCA in an offline simulator study. In: Proceedings of the driving simulation conference europe. Strasbourg, France, pp 101–108

Lanman D, Hirsch M, Kim Y, Raskar R (2010) Content-adaptive parallax barriers: optimizing dual-layer 3D displays using low-rank light field factorization. ACM Trans Graph 29:1–10. https://doi.org/10.1145/1882261.1866164

Levoy M, Hanrahan P (1996) Light field rendering. In: Proceedings of the 23rd annual conference on computer graphics and interactive techniques—SIGGRAPH '96. ACM Press, pp 31–42

Machover C, Encarnação M (eds) (2006) Tools and products. IEEE Comput Graph Appl 26:94–95. https://doi.org/10.1109/MCG.2006.24

Medina E, Fruland R, Weghorst S (2008) Virtusphere: walking in a human size VR "Hamster Ball". Proc Hum Factors Ergon Soc Annu Meet 52:2102–2106. https://doi.org/10.1177/154193120805 202704

Nahon MA, Reid LD (1990) Simulator motion-drive algorithms—a designer's perspective. J Guid Control Dyn 13:356–362. https://doi.org/10.2514/3.20557

Noma H (1998) Design for locomotion interface in a large scale virtual environment. ATLAS: ATR Locomot Interface Active Self Motion 64:111–118

Noma H, Sugihara T, Miyasato T (2000) Development of ground surface simulator for Tel-E-Merge system. In: Proceedings IEEE virtual reality 2000 (Cat. No.00CB37048). pp 217–224

Parrish RV, Dieudonne JE, Bowles RL, Martin DJ (1975) Coordinated adaptive washout for motion simulators. J Aircr 12:44–50. https://doi.org/10.2514/3.59800

Pölönen M, Salmimaa M, Häkkinen J (2011) Effect of ambient illumination level on perceived autostereoscopic display quality and depth perception. Displays 32:135–141. https://doi.org/10.1016/j.displa.2011.02.003

Reid LD, Nahon MA (1985) Flight simulation motion-base drive algorithms: part 1. Developing and testing equations, UTIAS

Reymond G, Kemeny A (2000) Motion cueing in the Renault driving simulator. Veh Syst Dyn 34:249–259. https://doi.org/10.1076/vesd.34.4.249.2059

Salmimaa M, Järvenpää T (2008) 3-D crosstalk and luminance uniformity from angular luminance profiles of multiview autostereoscopic 3-D displays. J Soc Inform Display 16:1033–1040. https://doi.org/10.1889/JSID16.10.1033

Schmidt SF, Conrad B (1970) Motion drive signals for pilot flight simulators. National Aeronautics and Space Administration

Souman JL, Giordano PR, Schwaiger M, Frissen I, Thümmel T, Ulbrich H, Luca AD, Bülthoff HH, Ernst MO (2008) CyberWalk: enabling unconstrained omnidirectional walking through virtual environments. ACM Trans Appl Percept 8:25:1–25:22. https://doi.org/10.1145/2043603.2043607

Venrooij J, Cleij D, Katliar M, Pretto P, Bülthoff HH, Steffen D, Hoffmeyer FW, Schöner H-P (2016) Comparison between filter- and optimization-based motion cueing in the Daimler Driving Simulator. In: Proceedings of the driving simulation conference Europe. Paris, France, pp 31–38

Venrooij J, Pretto P, Katliar M, Nooij S, Nesti A, Lächele M, de Winkel K, Cleij D, Bülthoff HH (2015) Perception-based motion cueing: validation in driving simulation. In: Proceedings of the driving simulation conference Europe. Tuebingen, Germany, pp 153–162

Watanabe H, Okaichi N, Omura T, Kano M, Sasaki H, Kawakita M (2019) Aktina Vision: Full-parallax three-dimensional display with 100 million light rays. Sci Rep 9:17688. https://doi.org/10.1038/s41598-019-54243-6

Weinbaum SG (1935) Pygmalion's spectacles

Wentink M, Pais RV, Mayrhofer M, Feenstra P, Bles W (2008) First curve driving experiments in the Desdemona simulator. In: Proceedings of the driving simulation conference Europe. Monaco, pp 135–146

Wetzstein G, Lanman D, Heidrich W, Raskar R (2011) Layered 3D: tomographic image synthesis for attenuation-based light field and high dynamic range displays. In: ACM transactions on graphics, p 11

Zhao J, Allison RS, Vinnikov M, Jennings S (2017) Estimating the motion-to-photon latency in head mounted displays. In: 2017 IEEE Virtual Reality (VR), pp 313–314

# Chapter 4
# Reducing Cybersickness

**Abstract**  VR may induce sickness effects because of visual incoherence between vergence and eye accommodation. These effects may be presented using convenient virtual screen distances in function of the used virtual world characteristics or appropriate light field technologies when the rendered objects are at distances which enact contradictory accommodation or vergence actions. However, a more difficult issue is navigation in the virtual world, when the user's movement is rendered visually yet not physically, which induces visuo-vestibular incoherence. The induced sickness effects need to be measured, and, if possible, predicted, to reduce the unwanted effects. Possible techniques include vibration seats, treadmills, and galvanic or auditory stimulation. The latter makes possible to modify the vestibular perception or at least reduce its weight in the sensorial fusion that the human brains perform. When producing physical, galvanic, or auditory stimuli is impossible, too costly or impacting user performance other travel techniques are proposed in this chapter, such as employing rendering effects under perceivable thresholds for the user. Furthermore, some recently proposed new technique are described, that use decomposition of movements, to prevent visuo-vestibular incoherence. Finally, the chapter includes an account of the practices to avoid VRISE based on its previously studied features and characteristics.

## 4.1  Measuring and Predicting VRISE

Motion sickness theories delve deep into the reasons behind VRISE. We saw in Sect. 2.3 that VR sickness originates from different factors. In this section, we review different methods to quantify cybersickness, before presenting strategies to alleviate its effects.

The literature is abundant on the topic and we want to report here the major methods that are commonly used. Cybersickness can be quantified in both subjective and objective ways.

### 4.1.1  Measurements Based on Subjective Features

Subjective estimation provides an easy-to-implement way to measure the level of cybersickness, as it mostly relies on questionnaires to fill out. Therefore, no specific device is needed. We present in the following subsections two questionnaires that are widely used in virtual reality and driving simulation: the Motion Sickness Susceptibility Questionnaire and the Simulator Sickness Questionnaire.

#### 4.1.1.1  The Motion Sickness Susceptibility Questionnaire

To detect susceptibility to motion sickness and, therefore, predict its occurrence in various dynamic environments, the Motion Sickness History Questionnaires (MSHQs) have been used for several decades to detect the kinds of motion that are most effective in causing sickness, one of the earliest and well-used versions being developed by Reason and Brand (Reason 1968; Reason and Brand 1975). An updated version of Reason and Brand's questionnaire was proposed by Golding (Golding 1998), and is now mostly known as the Motion Sickness Susceptibility Questionnaire or MSSQ.

The specificity of the MSSQ is that it is composed of two sections—one considering childhood experiences of travel and motion sickness before the age of 12, and the other considering experiences of travel and motion sickness over the last ten years. For each section, three tables are to be filled out corresponding to three questions: the frequency of travel or experiences with nine dynamic environments, the frequency of sickness or nausea feelings in these environments, and the frequency of vomiting in these environments. A formula is then provided to compute a raw motion sickness susceptibility score. A percentile conversion table is finally used (Golding 1998). A short version of the MSSQ also exists to cope with the limitation of the original version given by its length. The shortened version excludes the frequency of travel or experiences as well as that of vomiting (Golding 2006) (see Table 4.1). More recently, a Visually Induced Motion Sickness Susceptibility Questionnaire (VIMSSQ) was released from the MSSQ to specifically cope with Visually Induced Motion Sickness (VIMS) issues (Keshavarz et al. 2019). Therefore, rather than asking about past experience of travel and motion sickness, the VIMSSQ concentrates on the past use of visual devices (e.g., 2D/3D cinema, smartphones, TV sets, HMDs, simulators), with strong correlations observed between the reported level of VIMS and the nausea aspects of this questionnaire.

#### 4.1.1.2  The Simulator Sickness Questionnaire

When we look into papers related to immersion in virtual environments, and especially those dealing with virtual navigation, we quickly observe that researchers

**Table 4.1**  MSSQ-Short with the associated computation of the score (the table is the same for both sections—childhood and last ten years experiences)

| | Not applicable—Never traveled | Never felt sick | Rarely felt sick | Sometimes felt sick | Frequently felt sick |
|---|---|---|---|---|---|
| Cars | | | | | |
| Buses or coaches | | | | | |
| Trains | | | | | |
| Aircraft | | | | | |
| Small boats | | | | | |
| Ships, e.g., channel ferries | | | | | |
| Swings in playgrounds | | | | | |
| Roundabouts in playgrounds | | | | | |
| Roller coasters, Funfair rides | | | | | |
| | t | 0 | 1 | 2 | 3 |
| Raw score | $\dfrac{(total sickness score child) \times (9)}{9 - number of types not experienced as a child} + \dfrac{(total sickness score adult) \times (9)}{9 - number of types not experienced as an adult}$ The total sickness score is found by adding the score for each environment ("t" counts as 0) The number of types not experienced is found by counting the number of boxes in the "t" column Note that if the number of types not experienced is equal to 9 (none of the environments experienced), a division by 0 occurs, which implies the impossibility to estimate a participant's motion sickness susceptibility without any relevant motion exposure | | | | |

mostly make use of one method to measure sickness: the Simulator Sickness Questionnaire (SSQ). Proposed by Kennedy et al. (1993), this subjective method has quickly become the primary measuring tool for motion sickness and is now widely accepted in the immersive technology's community. According to Google Scholar, at the time of writing this chapter, there were more than 3200 citations for this tool—far more than other questionnaires.

The SSQ was primarily developed for aviation purposes—in particular flight simulators—and was built from former questionnaires and especially the Pensacola Motion Sickness Questionnaire (MSQ), which was itself built from previous questionnaires from the 1970s. It consists of a list of 16 items representing typical symptoms observed after virtual immersion (see Table 4.2). Participants are asked to rate each symptom from 0 (no sign) to 3 (strong signs). Each symptom is classified in

**Table 4.2**  Computation of SSQ scores

| SSQ symptom | Weight | | |
|---|---|---|---|
| | Nausea | Oculomotor | Disorientation |
| General discomfort | 1 | 1 | |
| Fatigue | | 1 | |
| Headache | | 1 | |
| Eyestrain | | 1 | |
| Difficulty focusing | | 1 | 1 |
| Increased salivation | 1 | | |
| Sweating | 1 | | |
| Nausea | 1 | | 1 |
| Difficulty concentrating | 1 | 1 | |
| Fullness of head | | | 1 |
| Blurred vision | | 1 | 1 |
| Dizzy (eyes open) | | | 1 |
| Dizzy (eyes closed) | | | 1 |
| Vertigo | | | 1 |
| Stomach awareness | 1 | | |
| Burping | 1 | | |
| Total | [1] $\times$ 9.54 | [2] $\times$ 7.58 | [3] $\times$ 13.92 |
| Total SSQ score = ([1] + [2] + [3]) $\times$ 3.74 | | | |

clusters: Oculomotor, Disorientation, and Nausea. The simulator sickness score is then computed according to a formula provided by Kennedy et al.

### 4.1.1.3  Critiques and Alternatives

The MSSQ is still considered as a highly reliable means to measure the susceptibility to motion sickness with high correlations with motion sickness ratings in the presence of motion stimuli (Golding 2006). However, Lamb and Kwok (Lamb and Kwok 2015) argued that Golding considered a too-small sample overrepresenting younger females, which might not be representative of the actual susceptibility in the general population. Although they do not question the questionnaire itself, they recommend choosing a sample that is representative of the general population in terms of age, sex, and even ethnic groups.

As for the SSQ, since its release, its reliability and applicability to VR were much questioned. For instance, arguments were made that exposure to VR leads to a different pattern of responses to the SSQ than with flight or driving simulators, implying that cybersickness may be different from motion sickness (Stanney et al. 1997). Among other criticism, Ames et al. (2005) regretted that the SSQ does not include enough optic-related symptoms, whereas VR makes an extensive use of HMD that can lead to strong optical symptoms. They also proposed that the SSQ be reduced to allow participants filling the questionnaire faster as cybersickness symptoms may decrease quickly.

Other arguments are that the assessment of the SSQ was realized only for military participants who were already predisposed to flight simulators, thus without proving its validity for people from the general population (Rebenitsch and Owen 2016).

To address the issues raised by the SSQ for an application in VR, several researchers suggested to revise or rescale the SSQ. For example, Kim et al. (2004) developed the Revised-SSQ (RSSQ) to fill some gaps in the SSQ such as the lack of important symptoms encountered in VR (facial pallor, vomiting) or the non-generalization to the general population. This revised questionnaire, however, is not commonly used in VR since no information on its validity is provided. Bouchard et al. (2007) revised the SSQ by excluding the Disorientation factor and changing the scoring for each symptom to better fit the observations done in VR. The corresponding revisited SSQ can be found online, with a translation in French.[1] This refactored version, though, seems not to be widely accepted, as the assessment was implemented on a population with a higher incidence of anxiety, which may have excluded other categories of people. Brucj and Watters (2011) tried to incorporate physiological responses in the SSQ, yet the methodology to validate the analysis was criticized (Stone Iii 2017). The CyberSickness Questionnaire (CSQ) was presented as an alternative to capture sickness symptoms typically arising in VR, taking nine items of the SSQ that would clearly indicate cybersickness while considering two factors—Dizziness and Difficulty in Focusing (Stone Iii 2017). Kim et al. (2018) proposed the Virtual Reality Sickness Questionnaire (VRSQ), employing nine items of the SSQ, considering Oculomotor and Disorientation factors only (excluding Nausea).

A comparative study was made to compare the SSQ and its variants for measuring cybersickness in consumer-oriented virtual environments (Sevinc and Berkman 2020). Results indicate that the SSQ is not applicable in commercial VR applications because of psychometric qualities, which is not the case with its variants such as the CSQ or the VRSQ.

Debates around subjective questionnaires for measuring motion sickness are interesting as they reveal the complexity of this phenomenon. All the proposed questionnaires derive from the SSQ, which is itself based on former questionnaires, indicating how powerful it is, since there has been no proposal for other radically different questionnaires.

A different approach was proposed by Bos et al. (2005), called the MIsery SCale (MISC). Rather than rating each sickness symptom from 0 to 3 as in the SSQ, the MISC proposes a single scale from 0 to 10, each point corresponding to a degree of "misery" that relates to the progression of the symptoms (see Table 4.3).

According to Bos, the MISC can be applied to any type of motion sickness (car, air, sea, space, VR) since it does not consider the possible underlying reasons for

---

[1]Laboratoire de Cyberpsychologie de l'UQO, Questionnaire sur les cybermalaises: https://w3.uqo.ca/cyberpsy/wp-content/uploads/2019/04/SSQ_vf.pdf.

**Table 4.3** Misery Scale (Bos et al. 2005)

| Symptom | | Score |
|---|---|---|
| No problems | | 0 |
| Uneasiness (no typical symptoms) | | 1 |
| Dizziness, warmth, headache, stomach awareness, sweating, … | Vague | 2 |
| | Slight | 3 |
| | Fairly | 4 |
| | Severe | 5 |
| Nausea | Slight | 6 |
| | Fairly | 7 |
| | Severe | 8 |
| | (Near) retching | 9 |
| Vomiting | | 10 |

sickness. The main advantage of this subjective tool is its great simplicity, as users need to give only one value, which—compared to the SSQ, requiring much more time and concentration—is very fast. However, the MISC focuses on nausea, whereas the SSQ also considers the oculomotor and disorientation effects.

#### 4.1.1.4   Questionnaires Administration

From the experiences in VR presented in the literature, questionnaires are usually administered before and after exposure to virtual environments. The simple reason is to get a baseline sickness score before exposure that will then be used to measure the extent to which a participant got sick or not during a VR experience.

However, although many researchers do not conceive doing otherwise, a few studies have demonstrated that this administration method is not correct and that questionnaires should be filled out only after exposure to VR. Indeed, first, Kennedy et al. (1993), to which most researchers in VR refer to, in their SSQ administration guide, explicitly do not recommend comparing scores between pre- and post-exposures. Second, a study conducted by Young et al. (2006) indicates that administering a questionnaire such as the SSQ prior to VR exposure can lead to biased post-exposure sickness scores (the authors measured an 80% increase when the SSQ was also filled out before exposure compared to when administered only after exposure). Explanations for this difference could be multiple: (i) asking participants to fill out a questionnaire on sickness effects may have a negative influence on their psychological state during VR exposure, as if they are required to answer to such questions, it may mean that the VR experience may indeed induce sickness, which lead them to expect becoming sick; (ii) participants may artificially report higher symptoms than what felt to satisfy the experimenter's expectations on the increase in sickness (Young et al. 2006).

Regardless of the administration method, people should be asked to fill out questionnaires just after exposure to virtual environments. Furthermore, they should be prompted to do so as quickly as possible to prevent them from providing responses that do not correspond to reality while wondering whether they feel or not such symptoms or the effects have diminished (Ames et al. 2005).

## 4.1.2 Measurements Based on Objective Features

Although questionnaires—especially the SSQ—are well established, they have one major drawback: they do not measure real-time sickness as they are generally administered after exposure to virtual environments. Some approaches to VR or driving simulation try to follow the evolution of sickness levels throughout participants' experiences by asking them to answer to one question at regularly spaced times (Nurkkala et al. 2012). The consequence is that participants may shift their attention away from their experience while focusing on their own sensations which may lead to biased results (Dennison et al. 2016). Furthermore, responses may be arbitrary (Katicic et al. 2015).

### 4.1.2.1 Software-Based Measurements

Other methods have been proposed that mainly rely on objective facts instead. For instance, the Motion Sickness Dose Value (MSDV) calculates a sickness value based on acceleration values. This metric was originally proposed for sea sickness measurements and was then adapted to cybersickness and named the Cybersickness Dose Value (CSDV) (So 1999). This value is computed as

$$CSDV = \int_{0}^{T} a(t)\mathrm{d}t$$

where T is the time of exposure to the virtual environment. As seen previously, this value depends on the user's actions and is measured from software.

### 4.1.2.2 Physiological and Behavioral Measurements

More popular objective measurement methods are based on physiological or behavioral aspects of the human body, such as Electrodermal Activity (EDA) (Yokota et al. 2005), Electrocardiography (ECG), gaze (Wibirama and Hamamoto 2014), Electroencephalography (EEG) (Kim et al. 2005), Electromyography (Aykent et al.

2012), heart rate variability, blood pressure (Holmes and Griffin 2001), Electrogastrography (EGG) (Himi et al. 2004), and postural sway (Takada et al. 2007) (see Sect. 4.3).

Electroencephalography measures brain activity through a cap mounted on a person's head on which electrodes are plugged. The measured quantity is usually the power spectrum obtained from the EEG signal. To analyze brain data, the signal is usually decomposed into several frequency bands called delta, theta, alpha, beta, and gamma (Sanei and Chambers 2013). Studies investigating changes in brain activity and more precisely, where and at which level changes occur under motion sickness conditions were conducted since the early 1940s (Jasper and Morton 1942). Although the subsequent experimental results did not reveal significant changes in brain activity, later studies reported that the power spectral energy in the delta band increases during motion sickness (Chelen et al. 1993). Furthermore, a significant positive correlation was observed between the cybersickness score as measured by subjective means and EEG delta wave, as well as a negative correlation between the cybersickness score and EEG beta wave (Kim et al. 2005).

Electrodermal activity, or skin conductance, measures the level of conductance between two points of contact on the skin and expresses the body's arousal level. It is measured through electrodes placed, for instance, on the palmar surface of fingers or the forehead. Past studies report skin conductance as an indicator of cybersickness. For example, changes in forehead skin conductance may quantify nausea (Gavgani et al. 2017). As cybersickness has a temporal effect (Stanney and Kennedy 1997), the rise of EDA is progressive by time, as the cybersickness level increases (Plouzeau et al. 2018). In contrast, in situations involving high cognitive loading events or inducing anxiety, the EDA can rise spontaneously (Wilson 2002; Di Loreto et al. 2018).

Physiological measurement techniques are interesting, as they can provide real-time indications on participants' state. However, most of them require intrusive devices, which may be uncomfortable for participants, thus affecting their psychological state. Fortunately, in the last couple of years, wearable sensors entered the market and allowed physiological measurements such as the electrodermal activity or heart rate, to be monitored in a non-intrusive fashion. One example is the Empatica E4 wristband[2] able to measure the evolution of EDA, the Blood Volume Pulse, acceleration, heart rate, and skin temperature.

### 4.1.3  Measuring VR Sickness Through Postural Sway Analysis

Among the presented objective techniques, postural sway retained the attention of several researchers in recent years. Indeed, following the theories of motion sickness exposed in Sect. 2.3 and especially the ecological theory, postural sway represents a

---

[2]Empatica: https://www.empatica.com/en-eu/.

natural behavior to follow during exposure to virtual environments. Previous research has found that postural instability precedes motion sickness (Stoffregen and Smart 1998). Postural sway thus represents a helpful metric to estimate VR sickness before it occurs and subsequently derives strategies to alleviate sickness effects. This feature is thus less constraining for users as it can be measured through totally non-intrusive devices, such as external cameras or balance boards.

Clinical studies using stabilometry measurements have considered parameters such as the area of sway, the total locus of the center of gravity and the locus length per unit area as efficient measures of the evolution of postural sway (Okawa et al. 1996). Their results indicate that the distribution of the center of gravity projected on an XY plane evolves from a dense distribution to a sparse one as participants are exposed to stereoscopic images (Takada et al. 2007). Based on these results, we present in this section further features to estimate VR sickness based on postural sway, and we provide insights on how to predict sickness.

### 4.1.3.1 Model of Postural Sway

Postural sway can be assimilated to the balance motion of the human body. By default, the human upright stance is unstable, as balance is achieved thanks to multiple flexible segments in the legs and the ankles. The brain continuously acts on the plantar flexors to keep the body upright, namely, without falling (Morasso and Schieppati 1999; Loram and Lakie 2002; Masani et al. 2003). A necessary condition for the body not to fall is to keep the projection of its Center Of Gravity (COG) within a zone called the stability area. Hence, postural stability can be defined as a stance with controlled—namely, voluntary—movements. Conversely, postural instability can be defined as a stance with uncontrolled—namely, involuntary—movements leading the body to fall down. From a motion sickness perspective, states with no signs of sickness are characterized by voluntary movements, whereas sick states are featured by an alternation between voluntary and involuntary movements (Chardonnet et al. 2017).

The balance motion of the human body can be simply modeled by an inverted pendulum (Masani et al. 2003). Figure 4.1 illustrates the corresponding model with the associated control-loop scheme. The input command is null as the goal is to keep the body in a quiet stance. Balance is regulated by the brain through a filtered Proportional-Differential (PD) controller. Several time delays are included in the model to reflect delays within the brain due to neural transmission and sensory-motor transmission.

### 4.1.3.2 Postural Sway Features

Simulation and experimental tests reveal several features of the postural sway that can be used to estimate cybersickness (Chardonnet et al. 2017). These features can be observed from the temporal domain as well as from the frequency domain of the postural sway signals.

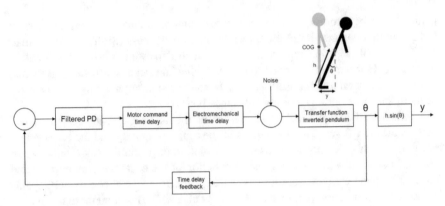

**Fig. 4.1** Closed-loop control for postural sway

As sickness occurs, the following events can be observed.

- The area on which the center of gravity projects (on an XY plane) grows;
- This area changes its shape, from an ellipse before the occurrence of sickness to a circle afterward;
- Frequency components of the postural sway spectra appear above 1 Hz;
- The difference between the post- and pre-exposures frequency components increases as the level of sickness grows.

Previous studies have shown that postural instability precedes motion sickness (Stoffregen and Smart 1998), therefore, these features could be used to predict cybersickness, as explained in the following subsection.

Although postural sway represents an important cybersickness indicator, past studies have also revealed that for seated situations such as driving situations, the correlation between motion sickness and postural sway may not be evident (Kemeny et al. 2015) and may be negative (Reed-Jones et al. 2008). Furthermore, a significant reduction in the incidence of motion sickness can be observed in seated positions (e.g., while playing videogames) when compared to standing positions (Merhi et al. 2007). This does not imply, however, that postural sway is not worth being measured in seated situations since the literature also provides evidence that body motion differs between users developing motion sickness symptoms and non-sick users in such situations (Stoffregen et al. 2000, 2008).

### 4.1.4   Cybersickness Prediction

From all the measurement methods described above, strategies to predict and avoid VR sickness can be derived. For instance, by monitoring in real time the features of postural sway, such as the shape and the size of the COG's projection area, and the frequency components of the postural sway signals, the sickness level can be tracked easily. When a change in the size and shape of the COG's projection occurs (or when frequency components appear above 1 Hz), users can be informed of possible risks in continuing being immersed, and the experience can be adapted accordingly. For example, speed or acceleration can be reduced or stopped in the case of navigation. Figure 4.2 illustrates an implementation example of a simple VR sickness predictor in a VR application based on postural sway measurements.

If the advantage of measuring postural sway is to avoid wearing intrusive sensors, its drawback is its difficulty in getting continuous measures without noise induced by the user's movements. The literature has recently provided ideas to predict sickness using postural sway measurements, but only in situations that are not specifically linked to virtual reality (Laboissière et al. 2015; Palmisano et al. 2018).

Alternatives to postural sway can be considered to predict VR sickness, such as head movements, through inertial sensors, and skin conductance. These methods, however, highly vary from person to person. Other alternatives are physio-behavioral parameters (e.g., heart rate and breathing) for which changes in the behavior indicate an occurrence of sickness (Kim et al. 2005). For example, Lopes et al. (2020) found out that more frequent eye blinks may be a sign a cybersickness, though no significant differences were spotted with non-sick individuals. Hence, we could imagine developing a VR sickness predictor based on physiological measurements: by defining a threshold above which the cybersickness level could become critical, adaptive strategies could be designed to keep users comfortable during their VR experience.

Another path to explore is artificial intelligence. With the highly increasing trend of machine learning and deep learning algorithms observed in the last years, artificial intelligence represents an interesting tool to predict the occurrence of VRISE. Indeed, if we can train the system to detect the sickness level, VR applications can include online strategies to adapt the VR experience so that the sickness level remains low. The major difficulty though is to get enough data to train the system. However, some perspective worth of investigation have recently been insightfully suggested (Wang et al. 2019a; Islam et al. 2020), with the possibility to predict cybersickness thanks to neural networks.

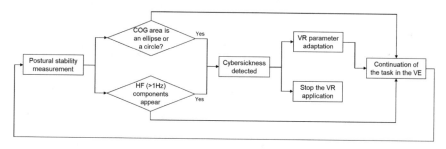

**Fig. 4.2** Example of a cybersickness prediction system using a postural stability measurement

### 4.1.5   Conclusion

Estimating cybersickness is a non-straightforward issue. Since cybersickness is a complex phenomenon, the means to characterize it are diverse with pros and cons for each of them. Table 4.4 summarizes the main ones. A common approach is to combine both subjective and objective means so that measures obtained from one method can be supported by the others.

## 4.2   Reducing VRISE Through Travel Techniques

One of the main factors inducing cybersickness is navigating in the virtual space using VR navigation devices rather than moving naturally, like walking. Cybersickness is

**Table 4.4**  Comparison table for estimating VR sickness

| Method | Pros | Cons |
|---|---|---|
| *Subjective* | | |
| MSSQ | • Predicts susceptibility to sickness based on past experience<br>• Long-standing questionnaire | • Long to fill out |
| SSQ | • The most common questionnaire in VR studies | • Long to fill out<br>• Initially designed for the aviation field, has had its validity to VR questioned |
| VRSQ | • Shorter than the SSQ<br>• More reliable than the SSQ | • Not much used |
| MISC | • Very fast to complete<br>• Suitable for any type of sickness | • Considers only nausea |
| *Objective* | | |
| MSDV | • No device required<br>• Easily computed | • Based on accelerations only and not on users' state |
| Physiological means (heart rate, EDA, etc.) | • Real-time measurement<br>• Representative of users' state | • May require wearing intrusive devices<br>• Some measures may not be reliable<br>• Need knowledge to analyze signals |
| Behavioral means (postural sway, etc.) | • Indicate the occurrence of sickness before it happens | • Real-time measurement hard to achieve<br>• Correlation with motion sickness not evident for driving simulation studies |

here caused by the conflict between visual and vestibular or kinesthetic stimuli (see Chap. 2, Sect. 2.3). Past literature provides an already well-furnished catalog of travel techniques to alleviate cybersickness effects. Hence, the need to develop new travel strategies mostly comes from the fact that physical boundaries constrain us due to technological and environmental limitations, which makes it difficult to navigate in potentially unlimited virtual spaces (Al Zayer et al. 2020). In these studies, travel techniques are evaluated not only for their ability to reduce cybersickness effects but also for their usability without generating high cognitive loads and their ability to ensure high levels of presence. Indeed, the primary challenge in designing navigation techniques is to simultaneously satisfy several criteria such as affordance—the ability of an object to suggest its usage—ergonomics, high levels of presence, and low levels of cybersickness. This challenge makes it hard to develop efficient travel techniques, as some of these criteria may conflict with each other (George 2016).

In the last few years, with the spread of affordable head-mounted displays, the trends have pointed to controller-based, teleportation-based, room-scale-based, and motion-based travel techniques (Boletsis and Cedergren 2019).

### 4.2.1 Teleportation-Based Techniques

Teleportation instantaneously transports a user from one point to another: a target is selected, and the user is automatically transported to this target (Bowman et al. 2005). At first glance, this technique seems intuitive, as it only requires pointing to the desired goal to travel in a virtual environment. Teleportation-based techniques thus represent an attractive alternative to travel in virtual environments and are now commonly used in many VR applications.[3] Furthermore, since no motion cues are perceived, they have been proved efficient in reducing cybersickness (LaViola 2000). However, an important limitation of teleportation is that it does not correspond to natural navigation and can cause a loss of spatial orientation (Bowman et al. 1997). Furthermore, in some applications, such as driving simulation or walking, when a vehicle or observer's behavior is part of the use case or the game, this type of solution is not applicable. More generally, past studies have demonstrated that techniques that do not allow users to control their movements (in terms of speed, acceleration, or view change) result in spatial disadvantages (Christou and Bülthoff 1999; Ragan et al. 2012). Several solutions exist to mitigate this effect such as.

- defining points of interest within the virtual environment so that, after teleportation, users are oriented toward the points of interest, or offering users to specify the desired orientation after teleportation (Bozgeyikli et al. 2016). Specifically, an arrow is displayed at the target indicating the direction that the user will be facing after teleportation;

---

[3]Teleportation is now a functionality included in game engines such as Unity or in VR platforms such as Steam VR, which facilitates and quicken its implementation in VR applications.

- animating teleportation: transitions from one point to another are implemented by interpolation with a constant (Bhandari et al. 2018) or variable (Mackinlay et al. 1990) speed. Animated interpolation can better maintain spatial awareness (Bowman et al. 1997; Rahimi et al. 2020); however, it induces high cybersickness levels, especially in the presence of rotational changes (Rahimi et al. 2020).
- introducing effects during teleportation, such as fading effects during transitions. For example, at the beginning of the transition, the environment fades to black, and it then fades back to normal at the new location at the end of the transition. This effect is used in videogames and is known as "blink" teleportation.[4] Although considered as robust, recent studies have indicated that such an effect does not lead to significant differences in terms of cybersickness levels with instantaneous teleportation (Rahimi et al. 2020).

### 4.2.2  Motion-Based and Room-Scaled-Based Techniques

As a compromise between real and virtual walking and in consideration of physical environmental constraints, several motion-based techniques have been devised to help maintain the feeling of walking naturally.

*Walking-In-Place* (WIP) is one of the first techniques proposed to induce head oscillations by requiring users to step in place (Slater et al. 1995). Many variants of WIP were later planned to capture people's movements and make them more natural. Specifically, they deal with motion detection with associated issues, such as kinematics, latency, occlusions, or the need for extra devices such as cameras or sensor platforms (Templeman et al. (1999), Fujita (2004), Feasel et al. (2008), Zielinski et al. (2011), Williams et al. (2011, 2013), Kim et al. (2012), Nilsson et al. (2013), Mirzaei et al. (2013), Guy et al. (2015)).

Dealing with walking naturalness and restrictions of physical space, Redirected Walking is a navigation technique that is gathering great attention, as it allows users to explore infinite virtual environments while walking in a real constrained physical space. This is made possible by taking profit of the dominance of the human visual system over the vestibular system (Razzaque et al. 2001). Specifically, the goal of redirected walking is to make users feel that they walk in a straight path, whereas they actually walk in a curved path in the physical environment. In practice, subtle rotational distortions, under detection thresholds, are introduced to redirect users to the virtual track. Several studies indeed rely for example on heuristics (Zhang and Kuhl 2013) or the prediction of the user's path in the virtual world (Nitzsche et al. 2004). The main question, which is the object of intense research, is to find the redirection gains that do not disturb users (Langbehn and Steinicke 2018), which involves determining the detection thresholds of the induced motion gains (Steinicke et al. 2008, 2010; Grechkin et al. 2016), as well as measuring the effect of gains on users performance and experience (Williams et al. 2006; Xie et al. 2010; Freitag et al.

---

[4]UploadVR, Cloudhead's "Blink" locomotion for VR is simple and robust, 2015: https://uploadvr. com/cloudhead-blink-vr-movement/.

2016; Ragan et al. 2017). An alternative to determining the right viewpoint rotations and translations gains is to act on the virtual environment's geometry using, for instance, self-overlapping architectures or the change blindness illusion to keep the user within the physical space (Suma et al. 2011, 2012). Another alternative, which has been suggested in CAVE systems, is to "reset" users' positions and orientations when approaching the boundaries of the physical space. These resetting techniques have mostly been developed to deal with the absence of walls in CAVE systems when physically rotating by applying rotation gains in a direction opposite the user's physical rotation for example (LaViola et al. 2001).

### 4.2.3  Controller-Based Techniques

Controller-based techniques involve control devices to travel in virtual environments. The most emblematic device is the gamepad, which embeds joysticks to control speed and orientation and buttons for further functionalities. Several controller-based techniques are presented as examples in the following. Current work is in progress at the Driving Simulation Association to investigate the deployment of such techniques in industrial applications.[5]

#### 4.2.3.1  Space Scrolling

*Space Scrolling* is a technique based on the use of a smartphone as the controller to navigate in a virtual environment. The rationale behind this choice lies in the strong familiarity with smartphones, as around half the world population holds a smartphone in 2020.[6]

The principle of this technique is rather simple: to move around, the user has to scroll his finger on the smartphone, as he or she would do to navigate on the internet. An effect of inertia is added to avoid sudden movements, such as infinite decelerations and sudden stop, which can induce a high level of cybersickness. In addition, the user is likely to move their finger several times on the screen to reach their goal, and the effect of inertia makes fluid movements possible in the virtual environment, thus preventing sudden jolts (George et al. 2013, 2014).

---

[5]Cybersickness, Driving Simulation Association: https://driving-simulation.org/cybersickness/.

[6]Statista, Number of smartphone users worldwide from 2016 to 2021, 2019: https://www.statista.com/statistics/330695/number-of-smartphone-users-worldwide/.

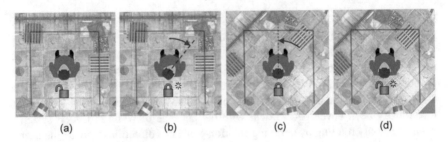

**Fig. 4.3** The *Head Lock* technique

### 4.2.3.2  Head Lock

Rotation is the part of displacement that is most likely to cause simulator sickness (Kemeny et al. 2015). *Head Lock* is a locomotion technique to optimize rotations (Kemeny et al. 2017) that can be combined with other travel techniques, as it mainly focuses on rotational movements. This technique can be seen as an extension of the *Grabbing The Air* travel technique (Bowman and Hodges 1997): the user turns their head to the desired angle, then closes one eye (Fig. 4.3b), which fixes the virtual environment to the head. When the user moves their head back to the front position, they perceive the virtual environment as frozen (Fig. 4.3c). Finally, they open their eye again to keep traveling (Fig. 4.3d).

### 4.2.3.3  Avatar Follow (Virtual Guiding Avatars)

*Avatar Follow* is a locomotion technique inspired by the *Path Drawing* travel technique (Igarashi et al. 1998) and *Space Scrolling*, described above. Following the same laws of motion as with *Space Scrolling*, the user moves an avatar in the environment (see Fig. 4.4). The system then automatically routes the user to the target position by modulating the acceleration as in *Path Drawing*. Early studies have claimed significant VRISE reduction when using virtual guiding avatars (Lin et al. 2004b), but recent studies are still to confirm significant sickness reduction effects.

Figure 4.4 includes an abstract representation of the avatar in the form of a semitransparent sphere indicating its position and a rod indicating its direction of translation. The sphere is placed at the height of the user's head to let them look in front of it while moving. When the user's position approaches that of the avatar, the sphere fades out so as not to disturb the user. Fading out occurs smoothly between 0.5 and 1 m. An arrow appears on the floor under the avatar so that the user can locate its orientation when the sphere is invisible. This is particularly useful when the user must initiate the move: the arrow is at their feet, and they can easily view and choose the direction. Motion is then performed considering speed and acceleration limits (see Sect. 4.3.1).

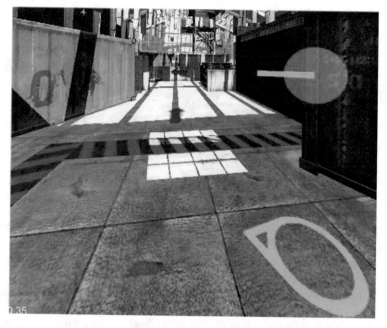

**Fig. 4.4** The *Avatar Follow* technique

### 4.2.3.4 Semi-Automatic Navigation

Techniques that do not allow users to control their movements result in spatial disadvantages (Christou and Bülthoff 1999; Ragan et al. 2012). An alternative to solve issues related to jerky movements induced by the use of controllers that lead to cybersickness effects takes inspiration from humanoid robotics domain, which has produced extensive research on path generation (Mohanan and Salgoankar 2018). One suggestion from that field is to provide hybrid navigation—namely, a mix between animated teleportation and manual control of navigation (Wang et al. 2019b). Specifically, users point their destination target either with a tracked controller or through gaze; the VR system then calculates in real time a path to follow that is optimized in terms of acceleration and jerk. Users are then free to either follow the path automatically as in animated teleportation or freely control their movement in terms of speed. Experimental tests indicate a decrease of cybersickness effects of about 34% with this technique.

## 4.3   Reducing VRISE by Adapting Existing Travel Techniques

An alternative to developing new travel techniques is to adapt well-established existing travel techniques.

### 4.3.1   Adaptation of Navigation Parameters

One way is to modify navigation parameters offline to reduce cybersickness. For instance, some studies propose recommendations in terms of navigation speed and acceleration to limit cybersickness, especially while using head-mounted displays and for applications linked to healthcare or video games (Porcino et al. 2017). So et al. (2001) indicate that from 3 m/s to 10 m/s root-mean-square, sickness symptoms and vection sensations increase but remain stable beyond 10 m/s root-mean-square. Interestingly, in the same study, it is observed that onset times of cybersickness can be significantly affected by navigation speed, with vection sensations manifesting earlier than nausea, which is not the case with the ratio between the increase of sickness and the duration of exposure. Recently, it was confirmed that low rotational accelerations ($2°/s^2$) yield lower cybersickness (Kemeny et al. 2015). Other studies consider the level of cybersickness as a function of the speed and the distance to a virtual obstacle such as walls (Mirzaei 2014): when users stand close (less than 1 m) to virtual objects, low speeds (under 2 m/s) are recommended. Oculus recommends navigation speeds that are close to real natural speeds—around 1.4 m/s for walking (Yao et al. 2014), as recently confirmed by Terenzi and Zaal (2020).

### 4.3.2   Adaptation Based on Field of View Reduction and Blur

On a different perspective, since the field of view is considered to be the main source of vection (Basting et al. 2017) (see Chap. 2, Sect. 2.2), several studies explore the effect of changing the field of view dynamically, based on the displacement on cybersickness levels (Fernandes and Feiner 2016). Results indicate that users are not bothered by this change; however, this usually applies to HMDs for which the field of view can already be quite narrow. Furthermore, the restriction of the field of view is mostly done from the center of the HMD, independently from where the user gazes at. As an example, eye gaze is considered to be always aligned with the head's position. Consequently, when a user has an eccentric eye gaze, peripheral optic flow can still be perceived, which may lead to VRISE. Adhanom et al. (2020) suggest considering the eye gaze position to move the center of the field of view restrictor accordingly, as they demonstrate it enables users to change eye gaze position more freely than when the position of the field of view is fixed.

An alternative to field of view reduction is blurring the scene while navigating. Previous studies suggest techniques to add artificial blurring, for instance during rotational motion (Budhiraja et al. 2017), or simulate the focus at a different depth to reproduce the depth of the field encountered in the human vision, thus enabling more realistic blurring (Hillaire et al. 2008). These techniques have proved to delay cybersickness onset of about two minutes without yet leading to a significant reduction of cybersickness levels (Budhiraja et al. 2017).

### 4.3.3 Adaptation Based on Users' Real-Time Physiological State

Another way of reducing VRISE is to adapt navigation parameters from the cybersickness level felt in real time by the user (Plouzeau et al. 2018). The idea behind this method is to demonstrate that without changing much well-known travel techniques—namely, without modifying users' navigation habits—cybersickness occurrence can be alleviated while maintaining navigation performance. Contrary to most navigation techniques where navigation parameters remain static since they do not depend on the user's state, navigation can be adapted as a function of the user's physiological state in real time. As we saw in Sect. 4.1.2, wearable sensors are now available that can measure the level of cybersickness in real time through physiological values, such as Electrodermal Activity (EDA): a progressive increase of EDA level means an increase of cybersickness level. Therefore, to prevent cybersickness from rising, one solution is to compute navigation accelerations as a function of the variation of EDA: when EDA increases, navigation accelerations decrease; conversely, when EDA decreases, accelerations increase. Both objective (e.g., Motion Sickness Dose Value, Electrodermal Activity, Postural Sway) and subjective (e.g., the Simulator Sickness Questionnaire) measurements indicate that cybersickness levels can be reduced by 71% by adjusting navigation (Plouzeau et al. 2018). Furthermore, measurements of cognitive load and navigation performance (e.g., total displacement of the users in the virtual environment, or quantity of actions on the navigation device) do not reveal any significant difference when adapting navigation to users, which means that the latter does not impact user experience (Plouzeau et al. 2018).

These studies show the interest of centering interaction on users rather than systems, conversely to what was mainly pursued in the past. More interestingly, this approach demonstrates that there is no specific need to change the whole world in terms of navigation techniques to alleviate sickness effects, as user experience can be enhanced by using existing navigation methods more smartly.

### 4.3.4   Techniques Using Salient Visual References

Several studies have suggested providing fixed references in the user's field of view to mitigate simulator sickness, such as a cockpit in a flight simulator, a vehicle passenger in a car simulator, or rest frames in virtual environments (Prothero 1998; Lin et al. 2002; Yao et al. 2014; Kemeny et al. 2017; Cao et al. 2018). This observation follows the rest frame theory explaining cybersickness and presented in Chap. 2, Sect. 2.3.4: cybersickness results from conflicting rest frames implied by many motion cues, which entails that observing stationary-looking objects such as the horizon conveys a stationary feeling of ground.

A variant of rest frames that attracted attention in 2015 to reduce cybersickness is to add a virtual nose (Whittinghill et al. 2015; Wienrich et al. 2018). Different from classical rest frames that are fixed relative to the world, the virtual nose is fixed relative to the head's position. Results indicate that time exposure to VR can be increased of about 94 s when there is no intensive rotational motion, while it increases of about two seconds when there is intensive rotational motion, which underlies that such rest frame may not be as efficient in critical scenarios involving intensive motion.

### 4.3.5   Other Adaptation Techniques

Argelaguet (2014) evaluated a speed adaptation technique where speed is adjusted as a function of the spatial relationship between the user, the environment, and the optical flow. The main drawback of this technique lies in the mapping between displacements from the device (a classical joystick) and virtual movements.

Sargunam (Sargunam et al. 2017) devised a semi-natural navigation method with amplified rotation factors. Though it proved to be efficient, their technique requires being seated, and its effects depend on users' past experiences.

## 4.4   Reducing VRISE Through Galvanic Stimulation

Early identification of electric sources in the human body by Galvani leads to using galvanic stimulation for health purposes, and when it was demonstrated that galvanic stimulation induces responses in the vestibular nerves (Goldberg et al. 1984), its employment to influence postural stability and orientation of motion spread rapidly (Bent et al. 2000). Subsequently, a visible effect of galvanic stimulation on vehicle control was demonstrated in driving simulation (Reed-Jones et al. 2007), identifying the possible role in simulation sickness reduction. The application of Galvanic Vestibular Stimulation (GVS) in fixed-base driving simulators to create vestibular motion cues and reduce motion sickness effects was thus presented.

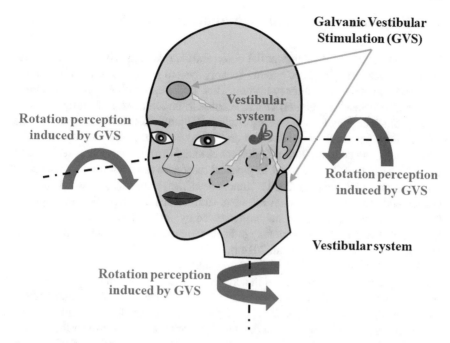

**Fig. 4.5** Illustration of rotation perceptions induced by Galvanic Vestibular Stimulation (GVS)

The effects of GVS on the semicircular canals (see Chap. 2, Sect. 2.1.2) provide a sensation of roll with a mild component of yaw through the combined effects of the stimulated canals (Fitzpatrick and Day 2004) (see Fig. 4.5). Several galvanic stimulation techniques were then proposed for industrial systems to reduce motion sickness[7] or provide motion sensations in VR.[8,9]

Unfortunately, the interindividual differences are often greater than the intraindividual variability, probably because of the perceived ambiguity of the unusual stimulation (MacDougall et al. 2002). Although several papers seem to provide evidence that galvanic stimulation may be an effective countermeasure to decrease simulation sickness (Cevette et al. 2012; Gálvez-García et al. 2015), effective implementations of GVS techniques are scarce. It would seem today that they will not be likely used in commercially available setups in the next future, as the used electric amplitudes are delicate to administrate without sufficiently stable results.

---

[7]Michael Cevette, Jan Stepanek, Anna Galea, Galvanic vestibular stimulation system and method of use for simulation, directional cueing, and alleviating motion-related sickness, 2014: https://patents.google.com/patent/US8718796B2/en.

[8]RoadtoVR, Samsung's New Headphones Trick Your Inner Ear to Move You in VR, 2016: https://www.roadtovr.com/samsungs-new-headphones-trick-your-inner-ear-to-move-you-in-vr/.

[9]vMocion: https://www.vmocion.com/technology.html.

## 4.5   Reducing VRISE Through Auditory Stimulation

The focus of previous chapters was the vision and the role of the visual system in eliciting cybersickness. However, another sensory system proved to actively contribute
to motion sickness: the auditory system. Past work reports that spatial sound can
elicit auditory vection when no visual, vestibular, or somatosensory information is
displayed, which may lead to sensory conflict (Väljamäe 2009). Vection can then be
significantly increased by reducing its onset time when auditory cues are added to
visual cues (Riecke et al. 2005; Keshavarz et al. 2014b). Furthermore, self-motion
perception can be influenced, too, as physical responses can occur in the presence of
spatial sounds (Tanaka et al. 2001). Nonetheless, the relationship between auditory
vection and motion sickness does not seem straightforward. In particular, empirical
research indicates that motion sickness induced by pure auditory stimulation arises
in some participants only, which may indicate the existence of an auditorily induced
motion sickness (Keshavarz et al. 2014a).

The driving simulation field, which shares substantial common issues (see Chap. 1,
Sect. 1.4), soon became interested in auditory stimulation as a means of alleviating
simulator sickness. Indeed, as described in Chap. 3 (Sect. 3.2), simulation without
any sensory stimulation (either visual or auditory) can lead to intense sickness, which
led researchers to develop motion cueing algorithms. A crucial aspect that gained
attention is the presentation of non-audible vibratory cues to reduce VRISE (vibrations and sounds being both waves but with different frequencies; see Fig. 4.6). In
fact, it is known that the human body is sensitive to vibrations depending on the
frequency, the amplitude, and the direction of excitation (Mansfield 2004).

Past studies indicate that adding vibratory stimulation can have a positive effect
on VRISE (McCauley and Sharkey 1992), but the choice of the frequency of the
vibrations is important since frequencies below 1 Hz make the user prone to sickness
(O'Hanlon and McCauley 1973). For instance, it was shown that 0.2 Hz represents
a translational oscillation frequency at which motion sickness is maximal (Golding

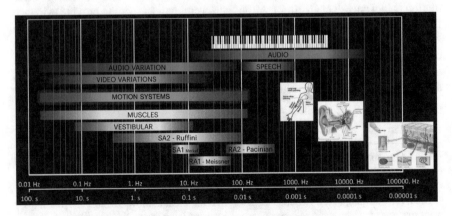

**Fig. 4.6**  Stimulation spectrum (courtesy of D-Box) (Maheu 2019)

et al. 2001). To alleviate VRISE, past works suggest applying high-frequency vibrations to the head (Bos 2015), which though may be highly disturbing in practice. The combination of loud (around 90 dB) auditory stimuli and vibratory (0.2–2 Hz) stimuli can restore postural stability (Nakajima et al. 2009), which, as described in Chap. 2 (Sect. 2.3) and in this chapter (Sect. 4.1.3), is an indicator of VRISE. More precisely, the quieter the auditory stimuli are, the more unstable the body posture is Nakajima et al. (2009). A study by Sawada et al. (2020) presents similar results by combining engine sounds from a motorbike engine emitting around 90 dB noises and vibratory stimulation whose frequency is modulated by the frequency of the sound: this combination effectively reduces cybersickness. Furthermore, realism is enhanced in the presence of sounds or vibrations, though sole vibratory or auditory stimulation seems to provide the best realism scores, which was also found in other studies (Plouzeau et al. 2013). Interestingly, the level of presence is not significantly affected by sounds or vibrations.

An alternative is to consider vibrations that affect proprioception and the vestibular system by applying vibrations in a range between 60 and 100 Hz, which can create the illusion of moving (Petroni et al. 2015). Recent studies indicate that implementing vibrations that either reproduce the vibrations felt in a real car (which usually range below 50 Hz and depends on the vehicle's speed or road granularity) or affect proprioception has a positive effect on VRISE (Lucas et al. 2020). However, the differences between both types of vibrations do not appear significant.

## 4.6 Best Practices for VRISE Avoidance

There are well-known rules and parameters to consider with a Virtual Reality (VR) installation to reduce cybersickness effects. Most of them are easily understandable or predictable from the data presented before. Their main parameters are listed in the following: a detailed description is instead provided in the preceding chapters and references.

### 4.6.1 Visuo-Vestibular Coherence in Navigation: Accelerations

As described in Chap. 2 (Sects. 2.2 and 2.3), one of the main cybersickness inducing elements are visuo-vestibular discrepancies induced by incoherent visual and physical motion cues. The most crucial cases are linked to accelerations above a perceivable threshold (Chap. 2, Sect. 2.1.2), especially when turning (rotational acceleration) while moving ahead. It is then mandatory to keep the acceleration levels below the human perception thresholds (horizontal and rotational when rendered only visually), or provide physical motion cues, thanks to motion platforms for coherent motion cues, or vibration setups to reduce vestibular information strength, or treadmills when walking.

The frequency of accelerations has also to be kept under a reasonable limit (see Chap. 1 Sect. 1.2.2), as their accumulation increases its Virtual Reality Induced Sickness Effects (VRISE). Furthermore, limiting acceleration onset values (see Otolithic organs, Chap. 2, Sect. 2.1.2) may protect from VRISE more efficiently than just limiting the corresponding acceleration values. To alleviate VRISE, high-frequency vibrations may be applied (Bos 2015), as it is supposed to reduce sickness due to lowfrequency motion (see Sect. 4.5), though may be disturbing in practice.

Finally, there are noticeable differences between users in reacting to visuo-vestibular incoherencies: some people are more sensitive than others (George et al. 2014). Hence, different VR setups can be implemented for two distinguishable groups of people: one group that is not very sensitive to cybersickness and the other group experiencing discomfort, stomach awareness, or oscillopsia (Allison et al. 2001) even with slight perceptual conflicts. Gender differences are also frequently reported in various VR studies (Holmes and Griffin 2001; Hakkinen et al. 2002; Flanagan et al. 2005; Häkkinen et al. 2006; Yang et al. 2012; Jaeger and Mourant 2016; Park et al. 2016).

Figure 4.7 illustrates the proportion of people experiencing VRISE as a function of stimuli intensity. This percentage increases when the intensity increases, but there will always be some people experiencing VRISE even before starting a VR experience, as well as others who will never suffer it. Cybersickness reduction techniques may change the shape of this curve, yet with little hope to get rid of VRISE for all users.

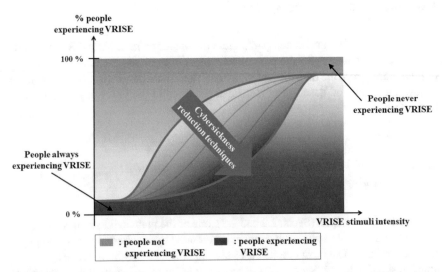

**Fig. 4.7** Illustration of the percentage of people experiencing Virtual Reality Induced Sickness Effects (VRISE) depending on the VRISE stimuli intensity. Cybersickness reduction techniques may allow the shape of the curve to be changed, yet some people will always experience VRISE just as some others will never do

## 4.6.2  Interactions and Control of Movement

There is a significant difference in experiencing VRISE when one is controlling or not the movement. As reported in Chap. 1 (Sect. 1.4.1), sensitivity to transport delay—the lag between (driving) actions and results in perceiving corresponding vehicle behavior modification—induces motion sickness and is significatively smaller for the driver than for a passenger who does not have efferent information on driving and thus cannot predict incoming movements. In the same way, when using navigational devices, such as joysticks, the provided displacement should be usual and predictable, at least after a learning phase, thus providing an internal model of navigation to the user.

## 4.6.3  Field of View

The Field Of View (FOV)—the instantaneous extent of the observed virtual world—visually represented by a solid angle, is one of the most impacting parameters in VRISE (Kemeny and Panerai 2003; Aykent et al. 2014; Kemeny 2014), as it influences the level of immersion and distance perception. Previous studies indicate that subjects consistently underestimate distances when using a wide FOV while overestimating distances with a narrow FOV (Kline and Witmer 1996; Knapp 2001). Nevertheless, whether impaired depth perception experiences in reduced FOVs are linked to the FOV restrictions or the lack of correct motion parallax information perceived in time while observing in limited FOV, is still debated (Creem-Regehr et al. 2005).

The field of view also influences speed perception (Jamson 2000), and a large field of view of at least 120° is required for correct speed perception in driving simulations. A sufficient large FOV is an essential visual parameter for correct speed perception (Kemeny and Panerai 2003), which can be explained by the differential speed perception role of central and peripheral vision (Brandt et al. 1973; Traschütz et al. 2012). These studies indicate that when the surrounding visual field moves around, self-motion perception depends on the peripheral stimulus, whereas, when observed only in the center of the visual field, the subject feels stationary with a moving surround (see Fig. 4.8; see Sect. 2.2 on optic vection in Chap. 2).

Consequently, various studies suggest a reduction of FOV to reduce motion sickness (see Chap. 4, Sect. 4.3.2). Indeed, in a small field of observation view, the conflict between perceived visual and vestibular motion is significantly reduced when turning—turning and rotational movements being among the worst cases for cyber-sickness. Conversely, when other factors, such as a substantial transport delay—namely, an overlong lag between an action and the rendering of its results—induce motion sickness, setups with a larger field of view may be preferred. A typical case is a stationary driving simulator with a large field of visual view, which may induce less motion sickness than a VR HMD (Aykent et al. 2014).

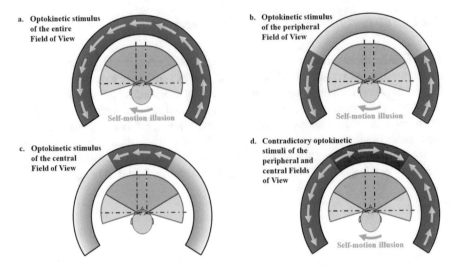

**Fig. 4.8** Influences of central and peripheral vision on self-motion perception. With a subject being at rest, a stimulus on the entire FOV (**a**) or the peripheral FOV (**b**) leads to apparent self-rotation. A stimulus on the central FOV (**c**) leads to the perception of being stationary in a moving surround. When stimuli on central and peripheral fields of view are contradictory (**d**), peripheral vision leads to apparent self-rotation

Therefore, field of view reduction is a largely proposed VRISE reduction technique (Bos et al. 2010; Fernandes and Feiner 2016), as it seems to be effective against motion sickness, though it strongly limits VR immersion level, and, consequently, rendering fidelity. Hence, this technique is rarely used with realistic and high-fidelity VR applications.

### 4.6.4   Latency

Transport delay—also called lag or latency—the VR system takes to respond subsequent user's actions, is one of the most critical parameters in VRISE (Uliano et al. 1986; LaViola 2000; Kemeny 2014; Wilson 2016) and may cause oscillopsia (Allison et al. 2001). Indeed, the delay between an observer's head motion and the resulting update on the visual display may induce not only uneasiness versus user's expectations but may also induce or reinforce conflicts between visual and vestibular information (see Chap. 2, Sects. 2.3.1 and 2.3.5). Though some papers report differences in transport-delay-induced VRISE between CAVEs and HMDs (Cordeil et al. 2017), they may also be linked to other factors, such as image resolution and immersion level (Colombet et al. 2016). Values of more than 70 ms for rendering lag cause perceivable cybersickness effects (Wilson 2016) and, for most HMDs, 20 or 30 ms[10] is considered as a target to avoid their effects for most users (Yao et al. 2014).

### 4.6.5  Duration of Exposure

Since the early use of VR, extended use of HMDs has been reported to induce cybersickness effects, stomach discomfort, nausea, and vomiting, especially during rotations (Bonato et al. 2009). We can cite the dismal failure of Nintendo's Virtual Boy,[11] unfortunately also experienced with Oculus, generated by head and display motions (Yao et al. 2014; Palmisano et al. 2017) some 20 years later. Duration of exposure is a critical factor, as it is directly proportional to its effects' strength and duration: the longer the exposure, the stronger and longer the effects (Kennedy et al. 2000; Yao et al. 2014). Interestingly, however, repeated experience of the same exposure, with a delay of several days between experiences, may provide resistance to simulator sickness (Domeyer et al. 2013), and taking breaks is advised in some cases (Yao et al. 2014).

Prior experience is also an essential factor (Chang et al. 2020), and gamers (see also Chap. 2, Sect. 2.3.5) or users with significant experience undergo much fewer sickness effects (George et al. 2014).

### 4.6.6  Independent Visual References

The presence of external visual references makes it possible to keep a stable world reference, which reduces VRISE (Prothero 1998; Jd et al. 1999). Visual immersion is also reduced when keeping external references, which reduces the potential conflicts between visual and vestibular cues. However, there is no limitation in providing full high-quality image rendering; hence, it is an efficient and often preferred technique. Several solutions and implementations were devised, including the virtual nose (Wienrich et al. 2018), initially introduced by a team of Purdue University.[12] However, the virtual nose, when used in HMDs, reduces VRISE only for a limited time. A display of a stable reference grid was suggested for CAVEs (Lin et al. 2002; Kemeny et al. 2017). Augmented Reality (AR) setups keep by definition external visual references visible, thus allowing low cybersickness effects. The latter are

---

[10] Adam Savage's Tested, The Challenge of Latency in Virtual Reality, 2013: https://www.tested.com/tech/concepts/452656-challenge-latency-virtual-reality/.

[11] Fast Company, Unraveling The Enigma Of Nintendo's Virtual Boy, 20 Years Late, 2015: https://www.fastcompany.com/3050016/unraveling-the-enigma-of-nintendos-virtual-boy-20-years-later.

[12] Purdue University, 'Virtual nose' may reduce simulator sickness in video games, 2015: https://www.purdue.edu/newsroom/releases/2015/Q1/virtual-nose-may-reduce-simulator-sickness-in-video-games.html.

mostly linked to visual discomfort or conflicts between vergence and accommodation (see below). However, optical see-through helmets are more efficient than video see-through setups, the latter composing computer-generated and camera-captured images, preferably with different image characteristics and lags in synchronization.

### 4.6.7  Binocular Disparity and Depth Cues

A well-known cause of visual fatigue that can induce sickness effects is linked to 3D display distortions in perceived virtual 3D structures versus real scenes as the 3D images are viewed on a display screen. Indeed, focus cues—accommodation and blur in the retinal image—specify the depth of the display rather than the various individual depths in the rendered scene (Hoffman et al. 2008). Additionally, the uncoupling of vergence and accommodation required by 3D displays frequently reduces one's ability to fuse the binocular stimulus and causes discomfort and fatigue for the viewer (see Chap. 1, Sect. 1.3.5). Light field technology is proposed to reduce the subsequent cybersickness effects, though commercially available systems are not yet available for everyday use.[13]

The beneficial effect of stereoscopy on distance perception seems to help the user (Perroud et al. 2020). This effect is still subject to ongoing research. Some authors report no effects in experiences lacking interocular distance calibration and head tracking for motion parallax in low immersive environments (Saracini et al. 2020).

### 4.6.8  Avatars

Early studies proposed a technique called *Virtual Guiding Avatar*, combining self-motion prediction cues and an independent visual background to reduce simulator sickness (Lin et al. 2004a). However, although avatars reduce discomfort, why they do so is not clear. Nevertheless, as the use of avatars is rapidly increasing in collaborative engineering and gaming, further studies may provide ample information on their role in reducing sickness effects significantly (see Chap. 4, Sect. 4.2.3).

The use of similar and progressively more and more high-fidelity avatars for own body rendering will increase the level of presence (Kilteni et al. 2012), and users will take avatars as an extension or replacement of their body (Botvinick and Cohen 1998; Ehrsson et al. 2005). Experiences in virtual environments confirmed this illusion (IJsselsteijn et al. 2006; Perez-Marcos et al. 2012); nevertheless, it was also demonstrated that a virtual hand may be dissociated in action (Kammers et al. 2009).

---

[13] Marc Levoy, Pat Hanrahan, Method and system for light field rendering, 2000: https://patents.google.com/patent/US6097394A/en.

Gamers, however, may get over this dissociation thanks to player–avatar identification, defined as a cognitive and emotional process (Li et al. 2013), and build a new operational extension of their body. Blending full-body tracking and gesture animation is now widely used in gaming. Still, differences between a player's actual and rendered movements (Bleiweiss et al. 2010) may pose a challenge in future industrial applications.

### 4.6.9  Ecological Setup and Experience

The ecological approach to visual perception, proposed in 1979 by Gibson (Gibson 1979), is a basis for well-adapted and efficient interface design for human–machine interactions for many (Rasmussen and Vicente 1989). Specifically, an ecological interface design can carefully analyze how the proposed VR setup can be used in the *affordable* environment of the user.

Many essential factors, such as ocular distortion correction or interocular distance measurements and calibrations, provide correct visual perception. For example, incorrect interocular distance may strongly affect distance perception, thus causing cybersickness. Another factor influencing distance perception is altitude (Panerai et al. 2001), which may induce cybersickness, in particular, when looking down or filling the field of view with the ground (Yao et al. 2014).

Finally, visual rendering levels, too, were reported as having an impact on cybersickness (Chang et al. 2020), which could be explained by the level of presence and by the impact of 3D cues if the visual richness is provided by an insufficient number of 2D textures, thus inducing false 3D cues.

Table 4.5 compares different VR devices, navigation techniques, and rendering techniques in terms of immersion, vision, and application. HMDs have been improved to minimize latency (Le Chénéchal and Chatel-Goldman 2018). Moreover, HMDs may lead to less vergence-accommodation conflict than CAVEs except for near objects observation, as accommodation is made at a constant distance of around 2 m. On the other hand, CAVEs can provide greater FOVs than standard FOV HMDs, as well as higher visual resolution (see Chap. 3, Sect. 3.1). Teleportation-based and controller-based navigation techniques can only partially consider visuo-vestibular conflict and users' expectations, depending on the used algorithm. Reduced FOV and blur techniques may reduce visuo-vestibular conflicts but also reduce immersion quality.

**Table 4.5** Comparison of different VR devices and navigation techniques, in terms of immersion, vision, and applications

| | Display technologies | | | | Navigation techniques | | | Visualization techniques | |
|---|---|---|---|---|---|---|---|---|---|
| | Standard FOV HMD | Large FOV HMD | CAVE | Light field Stereoscope | Teleportation-based | Motion-based | Controller-based | Visual references | Reduced FOV, Blur |
| *Factors relative to immersion* | | | | | | | | | |
| – Transport delay | +++ | | | | | | | | |
| – Observer's eye height | | | | | | | | | |
| *Factors relative to vision* | | | | | | | | | |
| – Visual integration of luminosity sources/Colorimetry | | | | | | | | | |
| – Vergence/accommodation conflict | +[2] | +[2] | | +++[3] | | | | | |
| – Field of View | | ++ ++ | ++ ++ | | | | | | |
| – Temporal and visual resolution | | | ++ | | | | | | |
| *Factors relative to application* | | | | | | | | | |
| – Visuo-vestibular conflict | | | | | ++[1] | +++ | +[1] | +++ | +[4] |
| – Expectations/Internal model | | | | | ++[1] | +++ | +[1] | | |

+ Taken into account/ ++ Expert configuration/ +++ Optimized configuration
[1] Partially taken into account/[2] Except for near objects observation/[3] Hardware prototype/[4] Reducing also immersion quality

# References

Adhanom IB, Navarro Griffin N, MacNeilage P, Folmer E (2020) The effect of a foveated field-of-view restrictor on VR sickness. In: 2020 IEEE conference on virtual reality and 3D user interfaces (VR). pp 645–652

Al Zayer M, MacNeilage P, Folmer E (2020) Virtual locomotion: a survey. IEEE Trans Vis Comput Graph 26:2315–2334. https://doi.org/10.1109/TVCG.2018.2887379

Allison RS, Harris LR, Jenkin M, Jasiobedzka U, Zacher JE (2001) Tolerance of temporal delay in virtual environments. Proc IEEE Virtual Rity 2001:247–254

Ames SL, Wolffsohn JS, McBrien NA (2005) The development of a symptom questionnaire for assessing virtual reality viewing using a head-mounted display. Optom Vis Sci 82:168–176. https://doi.org/10.1097/01.opx.0000156307.95086.6

Argelaguet F (2014) Adaptive navigation for virtual environments. In: 2014 IEEE symposium on 3D user interfaces (3DUI). pp 123–126

Aykent B, Paillot D, Merienne F, Kemeny A (2012) The influence of the feedback control of the hexapod platform of the SAAM dynamic driving simulator on neuromuscular dynamics of the drivers. Driving simulation conference. France, Paris, pp 377–380

Aykent B, Yang Z, Merienne F, Kemeny A (2014) Simulation sickness comparison between a limited field of view virtual reality head mounted display (Oculus) and a medium range field of view static ecological driving simulator (Eco2)

Basting O, Fuhrmann A, Grünvogel SM (2017) The effectiveness of changing the field of view in a HMD on the perceived self-motion. In: 2017 IEEE symposium on 3D user interfaces (3DUI). pp 225–226

Bent LR, McFadyen BJ, French Merkley V, Kennedy PM, Inglis JT (2000) Magnitude effects of galvanic vestibular stimulation on the trajectory of human gait. Neurosci Lett 279:157–160. https://doi.org/10.1016/S0304-3940(99)00989-1

Bhandari J, MacNeilage P, Folmer E (2018) Teleportation without spatial disorientation using optical flow cues. In: Proceedings of the 44th graphics interface conference. Canadian Human-Computer Communications Society, Toronto, Canada, pp 162–167

Bleiweiss A, Eshar D, Kutliroff G, Lerner A, Oshrat Y, Yanai Y (2010) Enhanced interactive gaming by blending full-body tracking and gesture animation. ACM SIGGRAPH ASIA 2010 sketches. Seoul, Republic of Korea, Association for Computing Machinery, pp 1–2

Boletsis C, Cedergren JE (2019) VR locomotion in the new era of virtual reality: an empirical comparison of prevalent techniques. Adv Hum-Comput Interact 2019:e7420781. https://doi.org/10.1155/2019/7420781

Bonato F, Bubka A, Palmisano S (2009) Combined pitch and roll and cybersickness in a virtual environment. Aviat Space Environ Med 80:941–945. https://doi.org/10.3357/ASEM.2394.2009

Bos JE (2015) Less sickness with more motion and/or mental distraction. J Vestib Res 25:23–33. https://doi.org/10.3233/VES-150541

Bos JE, de Vries SC, van Emmerik ML, Groen EL (2010) The effect of internal and external fields of view on visually induced motion sickness. Appl Ergon 41:516–521. https://doi.org/10.1016/j.apergo.2009.11.007

Bos JE, MacKinnon SN, Patterson A (2005) Motion sickness symptoms in a ship motion simulator: effects of inside, outside, and no view. Aviat Space Environ Med 76:1111–1118

Botvinick M, Cohen J (1998) Rubber hands 'feel' touch that eyes see. Nature 391:756–756. https://doi.org/10.1038/35784

Bouchard S, Robillard G, Renaud P (2007) Revising the factor structure of the Simulator Sickness Questionnaire. Annu Rev CyberTherapy Telemed 5:117–122

Bowman DA, Hodges LF (1997) An evaluation of techniques for grabbing and manipulating remote objects in immersive virtual environments. In: Proceedings of the 1997 symposium on Interactive 3D graphics. Association for Computing Machinery, Providence, Rhode Island, USA, p 35–ff

Bowman DA, Koller D, Hodges LF (1997) Travel in immersive virtual environments: an evaluation of viewpoint motion control techniques. In: Proceedings of IEEE 1997 annual international
symposium on virtual reality. IEEE Computer Society Press, Albuquerque, NM, USA, pp 45–52

Bowman DA, Kruijff E, LaViola JJ, Poupyrev IP (2005) 3D user interfaces: theory and practice.
Addison-Wesley, Boston

Bozgeyikli E, Raij A, Katkoori S, Dubey R (2016) Point & teleport locomotion technique for virtual
reality. In: Proceedings of the 2016 annual symposium on computer-human interaction in play.
Association for Computing Machinery, Austin, Texas, USA, pp 205–216

Brandt Th, Dichgans J, Koenig E (1973) Differential effects of central versus peripheral vision
on egocentric and exocentric motion perception. Exp Brain Res 16:476–491. https://doi.org/10.
1007/BF00234474

Bruck S, Watters PA (2011) The factor structure of cybersickness. Displays 32:153–158. https://
doi.org/10.1016/j.displa.2011.07.002

Budhiraja P, Miller MR, Modi AK, Forsyth D (2017) Rotation blurring: use of artificial blurring to
reduce cybersickness in virtual reality first person shooters. arXiv:171002599 [cs]

Cao Z, Jerald J, Kopper R (2018) Visually-induced motion sickness reduction via static and dynamic
rest frames. In: 2018 IEEE conference on virtual reality and 3D user interfaces (VR). pp 105–112

Cevette MJ, Stepanek J, Cocco D, Galea AM, Pradhan GN, Wagner LS, Oakley SR, Smith BE,
Zapala DA, Brookler KH (2012) Oculo-vestibular recoupling using galvanic vestibular stimulation to mitigate simulator sickness. Aviat Space Environ Med 83:549–555. https://doi.org/10.
3357/ASEM.3239.2012

Chang E, Kim HT, Yoo B (2020)Virtual reality sickness: a review of causes and measurements.Int
J Hum-Comput Interact 1–25. https://doi.org/10.1080/10447318.2020.1778351

Chardonnet J-R, Mirzaei MA, Mérienne F (2017) Features of the postural sway signal as indicators
to estimate and predict visually induced motion sickness in virtual reality. Int J Hum-Comput
Interact 33:771–785. https://doi.org/10.1080/10447318.2017.1286767

Chelen W, Kabrisky M, Rogers S (1993) Spectral analysis of the electroencephalographic response
to motion sickness. Aviat Space Environ Med 64:24–29

Christou CG, Bülthoff HH (1999) View dependence in scene recognition after active learning. Mem
Cogn 27:996–1007. https://doi.org/10.3758/BF03201230

Colombet F, Kemeny A, George P (2016) Motion sickness comparison between a CAVE and a
HMD. In: Proceedings of the driving simulation conference. pp 201–208

Cordeil M, Dwyer T, Klein K, Laha B, Marriott K, Thomas BH (2017) Immersive collaborative
analysis of network connectivity: CAVE-style or head-mounted display? IEEE Trans Vis Comput
Graph 23:441–450. https://doi.org/10.1109/TVCG.2016.2599107

Creem-Regehr SH, Willemsen P, Gooch AA, Thompson WB (2005) The influence of restricted
viewing conditions on egocentric distance perception: implications for real and virtual indoor
environments. Perception 34:191–204. https://doi.org/10.1068/p5144

Dennison MS, Wisti AZ, D'Zmura M (2016) Use of physiological signals to predict cybersickness.
Displays 44:42–52. https://doi.org/10.1016/j.displa.2016.07.002

Di Loreto C, Chardonnet J-R, Ryard J, Rousseau A (2018) WoaH: a virtual reality work-at-height
simulator. IEEE virtual reality (VR). Reutlingen, Germany, pp 281–288

Domeyer JE, Cassavaugh ND, Backs RW (2013) The use of adaptation to reduce simulator sickness
in driving assessment and research. Accid Anal Prev 53:127–132. https://doi.org/10.1016/j.aap.
2012.12.039

Ehrsson HH, Holmes NP, Passingham RE (2005) Touching a rubber hand: feeling of body ownership
is associated with activity in multisensory brain areas. J Neurosci 25:10564–10573

Feasel J, Whitton MC, Wendt JD (2008) LLCM-WIP: low-latency, continuous-motion walking-in-
place. In: 2008 IEEE symposium on 3D user interfaces. pp 97–104

Fernandes AS, Feiner SK (2016) Combating VR sickness through subtle dynamic field-of-view
modification. In: 2016 IEEE symposium on 3D user interfaces (3DUI). pp 201–210

Fitzpatrick RC, Day BL (2004) Probing the human vestibular system with galvanic stimulation. J
Appl Physiol 96:2301–2316. https://doi.org/10.1152/japplphysiol.00008.2004

Flanagan MB, May JG, Dobie TG (2005) Sex differences in tolerance to visually-induced motion sickness. Aviat Space Environ Med 76:642–646

Freitag S, Weyers B, Kuhlen TW (2016) Examining rotation gain in CAVE-like virtual environments. IEEE Trans Vis Comput Graph 22:1462–1471. https://doi.org/10.1109/TVCG.2016.2518298

Fujita K (2004) Wearable locomotion interface using walk-in-place in real space (WARP) for distributed multi-user walk-through application. In: Proceedings of IEEE virtual reality workshop. pp 29–30

Gálvez-García G, Hay M, Gabaude C (2015) Alleviating simulator sickness with galvanic cutaneous stimulation. Hum Factors 57:649–657. https://doi.org/10.1177/0018720814554948

Gavgani AM, Nesbitt KV, Blackmore KL, Nalivaiko E (2017) Profiling subjective symptoms and autonomic changes associated with cybersickness. Auton Neurosci 203:41–50. https://doi.org/10.1016/j.autneu.2016.12.004

George P (2016) Interactions nomades en environnement virtuel immersif pour des applications de revue de projet numérique. PhD thesis, Ecole Nationale Supérieure d'Arts et Métiers

George P, Kemeny A, Colombet F, Merienne F, Chardonnet J-R, Thouvenin IM (2014) Evaluation of smartphone-based interaction techniques in a CAVE in the context of immersive digital project review. In: The engineering reality of virtual reality 2014. International Society for Optics and Photonics, p 901203

George P, Kemeny A, Merienne F, Chardonnet J-R, Mouttapa Thouvenin I, Posselt J, Icart E (2013) Nomad devices for interactions in immersive virtual environments. In: IS&T/SPIE electronic imaging, the engineering reality of virtual reality. Margaret Dolinsky, Ian E. McDowall, Burlingame, USA, pp 86490I-1,86490I-7

Gibson JJ (1979) The ecological approach to visual perception. Psychology Press

Goldberg JM, Smith CE, Fernandez C (1984) Relation between discharge regularity and responses to externally applied galvanic currents in vestibular nerve afferents of the squirrel monkey. J Neurophysiol 51:1236–1256. https://doi.org/10.1152/jn.1984.51.6.1236

Golding JF (1998) Motion sickness susceptibility questionnaire revised and its relationship to other forms of sickness. Brain Res Bull 47:507–516. https://doi.org/10.1016/s0361-9230(98)00091-4

Golding JF (2006) Predicting individual differences in motion sickness susceptibility by questionnaire. Pers Individ Differ 41:237–248. https://doi.org/10.1016/j.paid.2006.01.012

Golding JF, Mueller AG, Gresty MA (2001) A motion sickness maximum around the 0.2 Hz frequency range of horizontal translational oscillation. Aviat Space Environ Med 72:188–192

Grechkin T, Thomas J, Azmandian M, Bolas M, Suma E (2016) Revisiting detection thresholds for redirected walking: combining translation and curvature gains. In: Proceedings of the ACM symposium on applied perception. Association for Computing Machinery, Anaheim, California, pp 113–120

Guy E, Punpongsanon P, Iwai D, Sato K, Boubekeur T (2015) LazyNav: 3D ground navigation with non-critical body parts. In: 2015 IEEE symposium on 3D user interfaces (3DUI). pp 43–50

Häkkinen J, Liinasuo M, Takatalo J, Nyman G (2006) Visual comfort with mobile stereoscopic gaming. In: Stereoscopic displays and virtual reality systems XIII. International Society for Optics and Photonics, p 60550A

Hakkinen J, Vuori T, Paakka M (2002) Postural stability and sickness symptoms after HMD use. In: IEEE international conference on systems, man and cybernetics. pp 147–152

Hillaire S, Lécuyer A, Cozot R, Casiez G (2008) Depth-of-field blur effects for first-person navigation in virtual environments. IEEE Comput Graph Appl 28:47–55. https://doi.org/10.1109/MCG.2008.113

Himi N, Koga T, Nakamura E, Kobashi M, Yamane M, Tsujioka K (2004) Differences in autonomic responses between subjects with and without nausea while watching an irregularly oscillating video. Auton Neurosci 116:46–53. https://doi.org/10.1016/j.autneu.2004.08.008

Hoffman DM, Girshick AR, Akeley K, Banks MS (2008) Vergence–accommodation conflicts hinder visual performance and cause visual fatigue. J Vis 8:33. https://doi.org/10.1167/8.3.33

Holmes SR, Griffin MJ (2001) Correlation between heart rate and the severity of motion sickness caused by optokinetic stimulation. J Psychophysiol 15:35–42. https://doi.org/10.1027//0269-8803.15.1.35

Igarashi T, Kadobayashi R, Mase K, Tanaka H (1998) Path drawing for 3D walkthrough. In: Proceedings of the 11th annual ACM symposium on user interface software and technology. Association for Computing Machinery, San Francisco, California, USA, pp 173–174

IJsselsteijn WA, de Kort YAW, Haans A (2006) Is this my hand i see before me? the rubber hand illusion in reality, virtual reality, and mixed reality. Presence: Teleoperators Virtual Environ 15:455–464 . https://doi.org/https://doi.org/10.1162/pres.15.4.455

Islam R, Lee Y, Jaloli M, Muhammad I, Zhu D, Quarles J (2020) Automatic detection of cybersickness from physiological signal in a virtual roller coaster simulation. In: IEEE VR

Jaeger BK, Mourant RR (2016)Comparison of simulator sickness using static and dynamic walking simulators. In: Proceedings of the human factors and ergonomics society annual meeting.https://doi.org/10.1177/154193120104502709

Jamson H (2000) Driving simulation validity: issues of field of view and resolution. In: Proceedings of the driving simulation conference. pp 57–64

Jasper HH, Morton G (1942) Electroencephalography in relation to motion sickness in volunteers. In: Proceedings of the conference on motion sickness. national research council of Canada

Prothero JD, Draper MH, Furness 3rd TA, Parker DE, Wells MJ (1999)The use of an independent visual background to reduce simulator side-effects.Aviat Space Environ Med 70:277–283

Kammers MPM, de Vignemont F, Verhagen L, Dijkerman HC (2009) The rubber hand illusion in action. Neuropsychologia 47:204–211. https://doi.org/10.1016/j.neuropsychologia.2008.07.028

Katicic J, Häfner P, Ovtcharova J (2015) Methodology for emotional assessment of product design by customers in virtual reality. Presence: Teleoperators Virtual Environ 24:62–73. https://doi.org/https://doi.org/10.1162/PRES_a_00215

Kemeny A (2014) From driving simulation to virtual reality. In: Proceedings of the 2014 virtual reality international conference. Association for Computing Machinery, Laval, France, pp 1–5

Kemeny A, Colombet F, Denoual T (2015) How to avoid simulation sickness in virtual environments during user displacement. In: The engineering reality of virtual reality 2015. International Society for Optics and Photonics, p 939206

Kemeny A, George P, Mérienne F, Colombet F (2017) New vr navigation techniques to reduce cybersickness. Electron Imaging 2017:48–53

Kemeny A, Panerai F (2003) Evaluating perception in driving simulation experiments. Trends Cogn Sci 7:31–37. https://doi.org/10.1016/S1364-6613(02)00011-6

Kennedy RS, Lane NE, Berbaum KS, Lilienthal MG (1993) Simulator Sickness Questionnaire: an enhanced method for quantifying simulator sickness. Int J Aviat Psychol 3:203–220. https://doi.org/https://doi.org/10.1207/s15327108ijap0303_3

Kennedy RS, Stanney KM, Dunlap WP (2000) Duration and exposure to virtual environments: sickness curves during and across sessions. Presence: Teleoperators Virtual Environ 9:463–472

Keshavarz B, Hettinger LJ, Kennedy RS, Campos JL (2014) Demonstrating the potential for dynamic auditory stimulation to contribute to motion sickness. PLoS ONE 9:e101016. https://doi.org/10.1371/journal.pone.0101016

Keshavarz B, Hettinger LJ, Vena D, Campos JL (2014) Combined effects of auditory and visual cuesErreur ! Signet non défini. on the perception of vection. Exp Brain Res 232:827–836

Keshavarz B, Saryazdi R, Campos JL, Golding JF (2019)Introducing the VIMSSQ: measuring susceptibility to visually induced motion sickness. In: Proceedings of the human factors and ergonomics society annual meeting.https://doi.org/10.1177/1071181319631216

Kilteni K, Groten R, Slater M (2012) The sense of embodiment in virtual reality. Presence: Teleoperators Virtual Environ 21:373–387 . https://doi.org/https://doi.org/10.1162/PRES_a_00124

Kim DH, Parker DE, Park MY (2004) A new procedure for measuring simulator sickness–the RSSQ

Kim HK, Park J, Choi Y, Choe M (2018) Virtual reality sickness questionnaire (VRSQ): motion sickness measurement index in a virtual reality environment. Appl Ergon 69:66–73. https://doi.org/10.1016/j.apergo.2017.12.016

Kim J-S, Gračanin D, Quek F (2012) Sensor-fusion walking-in-place interaction technique using mobile devices. In: 2012 IEEE virtual reality workshops (VRW). pp 39–42

Kim YY, Kim HJ, Kim EN, Ko HD, Kim HT (2005) Characteristic changes in the physiological components of cybersickness. Psychophysiology 42:616–625. https://doi.org/10.1111/j.1469-8986.2005.00349.x

Kline PB, Witmer BG (1996) Distance perception in virtual environments: effects of field of view and surface texture at near distances. Proc Hum Factors Ergon Soc Annu Meet 40:1112–1116. https://doi.org/10.1177/154193129604002201

Knapp JM (2001) The visual perception of egocentric distance in virtual environments. ProQuest Information & Learning

Laboissière R, Letievant J-C, Ionescu E, Barraud P-A, Mazzuca M, Cian C (2015) Relationship between spectral characteristics of spontaneous postural sway and motion sickness susceptibility. PLoS ONE 10:e0144466. https://doi.org/10.1371/journal.pone.0144466

Lamb S, Kwok KCS (2015) MSSQ-short norms may underestimate highly susceptible individuals: updating the MSSQ-short norms. Hum Factors 57:622–633. https://doi.org/10.1177/0018720814555862

Langbehn E, Steinicke F (2018) Redirected walking in virtual reality. In: Lee N (ed) Encyclopedia of computer graphics and games. Springer International Publishing, Cham, pp 1–11

LaViola JJ (2000) A discussion of cybersickness in virtual environments. SIGCHI Bull 32:47–56

LaViola JJ, Feliz DA, Keefe DF, Zeleznik RC (2001) Hands-free multi-scale navigation in virtual environments. In: Proceedings of the 2001 symposium on Interactive 3D graphics. Association for Computing Machinery, New York, NY, USA, pp 9–15

Le Chénéchal M, Chatel-Goldman J (2018) HTC Vive Pro time performance benchmark for scientific research. In: ICAT-EGVE 2018. Limassol, Cyprus

Li DD, Liau AK, Khoo A (2013) Player-Avatar Identification in video gaming: concept and measurement. Comput Hum Behav 29:257–263. https://doi.org/10.1016/j.chb.2012.09.002

Lin JJ, Abi-Rached H, Lahav M (2004a) Virtual guiding avatar: An effective procedure to reduce simulator sickness in virtual environments. In: Proceedings of the SIGCHI conference on Human factors in computing systems. pp 719–726

Lin JJW, Abi-Rached H, Lahav M (2004b) Virtual guiding avatar: an effective procedure to reduce simulator sickness in virtual environments. In: Proceedings of the SIGCHI conference on human factors in computing systems. Association for Computing Machinery, Vienna, Austria, pp 719–726

Lin JJ-W, Abi-Rached H, Kim D-H, Parker DE, Furness TA (2002) A "Natural" independent visual background reduced simulator sickness. Proc Hum Factors Ergon Soc Annu Meet 46:2124–2128. https://doi.org/10.1177/154193120204602605

Lopes P, Tian N, Boulic R (2020) Exploring blink-rate behaviors for cybersickness detection in VR. In: IEEE VR

Loram ID, Lakie M (2002) Direct measurement of human ankle stiffness during quiet standing: the intrinsic mechanical stiffness is insufficient for stability. J Phys 545:1041–1053. https://doi.org/10.1113/jphysiol.2002.025049

Lucas G, Kemeny A, Paillot D, Colombet F (2020) A simulation sickness study on a driving simulator equipped with a vibration platform. Transp Res Part F: Traffic Psychol Behav 68:15–22. https://doi.org/10.1016/j.trf.2019.11.011

MacDougall HG, Brizuela AE, Burgess AM, Curthoys IS (2002) Between-subject variability and within-subject reliability of the human eye-movement response to bilateral galvanic (DC) vestibular stimulation. Exp Brain Res 144:69–78. https://doi.org/10.1007/s00221-002-1038-4

Mackinlay JD, Card SK, Robertson GG (1990) Rapid controlled movement through a virtual 3D workspace. In: Proceedings of the 17th annual conference on computer graphics and interactive techniques. Association for Computing Machinery, Dallas, TX, USA, pp 171–176

Maheu V (2019) The art & sciences behinf creating immersive whole-body experiences

Mansfield NJ (2004) Human response to vibration. CRC Press

Masani K, Popovic MR, Nakazawa K, Kouzaki M, Nozaki D (2003) Importance of body sway velocity information in controlling ankle extensor activities during quiet stance. J Neurophysiol 90:3774–3782. https://doi.org/10.1152/jn.00730.2002

McCauley ME, Sharkey TJ (1992) Cybersickness: perception of self-motion in virtual environments. Presence: Teleoperators Virtual Environ 1:311–318 . https://doi.org/https://doi.org/10.1162/pres. 1992.1.3.311

Merhi O, Faugloire E, Flanagan M, Stoffregen TA (2007) Motion sickness, console video games, and head-mounted displays. Hum Factors 49:920–934. https://doi.org/10.1518/001872007X23 0262

Mirzaei MA (2014) Influence of interaction techniques on VIMS in virtual environments: estimation and prediction. PhD thesis, Ecole Nationale Supérieure d'Arts et Métiers

Mirzaei MA, Chardonnet J-R, Père C, Merienne F (2013) Improvement of the real-time gesture analysis by a new mother wavelet and the application for the navigation inside a scale-one 3D system. IEEE international conference on advanced video and signal-based surveillance. Krakow, Poland, pp 270–275

Mohanan MG, Salgoankar A (2018) A survey of robotic motion planning in dynamic environments. Robot Auton Syst 100:171–185. https://doi.org/10.1016/j.robot.2017.10.011

Morasso PG, Schieppati M (1999) Can muscle stiffness alone stabilize upright standing? J Neurophysiol 82:1622–1626. https://doi.org/10.1152/jn.1999.82.3.1622

Nakajima S, Ino S, Kazuhiko Yamashita, Mitsuru Sato, Akio Kimura (2009) Proposal of reduction method of mixed reality sickness using auditory stimuli for advanced driver assistance systems. In: 2009 IEEE international conference on industrial technology. pp 1–5

Nilsson NC, Serafin S, Laursen MH, Pedersen KS, Sikström E, Nordahl R (2013) Tapping-In-Place: increasing the naturalness of immersive walking-in-place locomotion through novel gestural input. In: 2013 IEEE symposium on 3D user interfaces (3DUI). pp 31–38

Nitzsche N, Hanebeck UD, Schmidt G (2004) Motion compression for telepresent walking in large target environments. Presence: Teleoperators Virtual Environ 13:44–60 . https://doi.org/https:// doi.org/10.1162/105474604774048225

Nurkkala V-M, Koskela K, Kalermo J, Nevanperä S, Järvilehto T (2012) A method to evaluate temporal appearances of simulator sickness during driving simulation experiments. Driving simulation conference. France, Paris, pp 41–49

O'Hanlon JF, McCauley ME (1973) Motion sickness incidence as a function of the frequency and acceleration of vertical sinusoidal motion. Canyon Research Group Inc Goleta Ca Human Factors Research Div

Okawa T, Tokita T, Shibata Y, Ogawa T, Miyata H (1996) Stabilometry-significance of locus length per unit area (L/A) in patients with equilibrium disturbances. Equilib Res 55:283–293. https:// doi.org/10.3757/jser.55.283

Palmisano S, Arcioni B, Stapley PJ (2018) Predicting vection and visually induced motion sickness based on spontaneous postural activity. Exp Brain Res 236:315–329. https://doi.org/10.1007/s00 221-017-5130-1

Palmisano S, Mursic R, Kim J (2017) Vection and cybersickness generated by head-and-display motion in the Oculus Rift. Displays 46:1–8. https://doi.org/10.1016/j.displa.2016.11.001

Panerai F, Droulez J, Kelada J-M, Kemeny A, Balligand E, Favre B (2001) Speed and safety distance control in truck driving: comparison of simulation and real-world environment. In: Proceedings of the driving simulation conference

Park GD, Allen RW, Fiorentino D, Rosenthal TJ, Cook ML (2016)Simulator sickness scores according to symptom susceptibility, age, and gender for an older driver assessment study. In: Proceedings of the human factors and ergonomics society annual meeting.https://doi.org/10.1177/ 154193120605002607

Perez-Marcos D, Sanchez-Vives MV, Slater M (2012) Is my hand connected to my body? The impact of body continuity and arm alignment on the virtual hand illusion. Cogn Neurodyn 6:295–305. https://doi.org/10.1007/s11571-011-9178-5

Perroud B, Gosson R, Colombet F, Regnier S, Collinet J-C, Kemeny A (2020) Contribution of stereoscopy and motion parallax for inter-vehicular distance estimation in driving simulator experiments. In: Proceedings of the driving simulation conference 2020 Europe VR. Driving Simulation Association

Petroni A, Carbajal MJ, Sigman M (2015) Proprioceptive body illusions modulate the visual perception of reaching distance. PLoS ONE 10:e0131087. https://doi.org/10.1371/journal.pone.0131087

Plouzeau J, Chardonnet J-R, Merienne F (2018) Using cybersickness indicators to adapt navigation in virtual reality: a pre-study. In: 2018 IEEE conference on virtual reality and 3D user interfaces (VR). pp 661–662

Plouzeau J, Paillot D, Aykent B, Merienne F (2013) Vibrations in dynamic driving simulator: study and implementation. In: Conference. Biarritz, France

Porcino TM, Clua E, Trevisan D, Vasconcelos CN, Valente L (2017) Minimizing cyber sickness in head mounted display systems: design guidelines and applications. 2017 IEEE 5th international conference on serious games and applications for health (SeGAH). IEEE, Perth, Australia, pp 1–6

Prothero JD (1998) The role of rest frames in vection, presence and motion sickness. PhD Thesis, University of Washington, HIT-Lab

Ragan ED, Scerbo S, Bacim F, Bowman DA (2017) Amplified head rotation in virtual reality and the effects on 3D search, training transfer, and spatial orientation. IEEE Trans Vis Comput Graph 23:1880–1895. https://doi.org/10.1109/TVCG.2016.2601607

Ragan ED, Wood A, McMahan RP, Bowman DA (2012) Trade-offs related to travel techniques and level of display fidelity in virtual data-analysis environments. In: Joint virtual reality conference of ICAT - EGVE - EuroVR. The Eurographics Association

Rahimi K, Banigan C, Ragan ED (2020) Scene transitions and teleportation in virtual reality and the implications for spatial awareness and sickness. IEEE Trans Vis Comput Graph 26:2273–2287. https://doi.org/10.1109/TVCG.2018.2884468

Rasmussen J, Vicente KJ (1989) Coping with human errors through system design: implications for ecological interface design. Int J Man Mach Stud 31:517–534. https://doi.org/10.1016/0020-7373(89)90014-X

Razzaque S, Kohn Z, Whitton MC (2001) Redirected walking. In: Proceeedings of eurographics. pp 105–106

Reason JT (1968) Relations between motion sickness susceptibility, the spiral after-effect and loudness estimation. Br J Psychol 59:385–393. https://doi.org/10.1111/j.2044-8295.1968.tb01153.x

Reason JT, Brand JJ (1975) Motion sickness. Academic Press, Oxford, England

Rebenitsch L, Owen C (2016) Review on cybersickness in applications and visual displays. Virtual Rity 20:101–125. https://doi.org/10.1007/s10055-016-0285-9

Reed-Jones RJ, Reed-Jones BH, Trick LM, Vallis LA (2007) Can galvanic vestibular stimulation reduce simulator adaptation syndrome? Driv Assess Conf 4:534–540

Reed-Jones RJ, Vallis LA, Reed-Jones JG, Trick LM (2008) The relationship between postural stability and virtual environment adaptation. Neurosci Lett 435:204–209. https://doi.org/10.1016/j.neulet.2008.02.047

Riecke BE, Schulte-Pelkum J, Caniard F, Bülthoff HH (2005) Influence of auditory cues on the visually-induced self-motion illusion (Circular Vection) in virtual reality. University College London, pp 49–57

Sanei S, Chambers JA (2013) EEG signal processing. Wiley

Saracini C, Basso D, Olivetti Belardinelli M (2020) Stereoscopy does not improve metric distance estimations in virtual environments. In: Cicalò E (ed) Proceedings of the 2nd international and interdisciplinary conference on image and imagination. Springer International Publishing, Cham, pp 907–922

Sargunam SP, Moghadam KR, Suhail M, Ragan ED (2017) Guided head rotation and amplified head rotation: evaluating semi-natural travel and viewing techniques in virtual reality. In: 2017 IEEE virtual reality (VR). pp 19–28

Sawada Y, Itaguchi Y, Hayashi M, Aigo K, Miyagi T, Miki M, Kimura T, Miyazaki M (2020) Effects of synchronised engine sound and vibration presentation on visually induced motion sickness. Sci Rep 10:7553. https://doi.org/10.1038/s41598-020-64302-y

Sevinc V, Berkman MI (2020) Psychometric evaluation of Simulator Sickness Questionnaire and its variants as a measure of cybersickness in consumer virtual environments. Appl Ergon 82:102958. https://doi.org/10.1016/j.apergo.2019.102958

Slater M, Steed A, Usoh M (1995) The virtual treadmill: a naturalistic metaphor for navigation in immersive virtual environments. In: Göbel M (ed) Virtual environments '95. Springer, Vienna, pp 135–148

So RHY (1999) The search for a cybersickness dose value. In: Proceedings of HCI international (the 8th international conference on human-computer interaction) on human-computer interaction: ergonomics and user interfaces-volume i - volume I. L. Erlbaum Associates Inc., USA, pp 152–156

So RHY, Lo WT, Ho ATK (2001) Effects of navigation speed on motion sickness caused by an immersive virtual environment. Hum Factors 43:452–461. https://doi.org/10.1518/001872001 775898223

Stanney KM, Kennedy RS (1997) The psychometrics of cybersickness. Commun ACM 40:66–69

Stanney KM, Kennedy RS, Drexler JM (1997) Cybersickness is Not Simulator Sickness. Proc Hum Factors Ergon Soc Annu Meet 41:1138–1142. https://doi.org/10.1177/107118139704100292

Steinicke F, Bruder G, Jerald J, Frenz H, Lappe M (2008) Analyses of human sensitivity to redirected walking. In: Proceedings of the 2008 ACM symposium on virtual reality software and technology. Association for Computing Machinery, Bordeaux, France, pp 149–156

Steinicke F, Bruder G, Jerald J, Frenz H, Lappe M (2010) Estimation of detection thresholds for redirected walking techniques. IEEE Trans Vis Comput Graph 16:17–27. https://doi.org/10.1109/TVCG.2009.62

Stoffregen TA, Smart LJ (1998) Postural instability precedes motion sickness. Brain Res Bull 47:437–448. https://doi.org/10.1016/S0361-9230(98)00102-6

Stoffregen TA, Faugloire E, Yoshida K, Flanagan MB, Merhi O (2008) Motion sickness and postural sway in console video games. Hum Factors 50:322–331. https://doi.org/10.1518/001872008X25 0755

Stoffregen TA, Hettinger LJ, Haas MW, Roe MM, Smart LJ (2000) Postural instability and motion sickness in a fixed-base flight simulator. Hum Factors 42:458–469. https://doi.org/10.1518/001 872000779698097

Stone Iii W (2017) Psychometric evaluation of the simulator sickness questionnaire as a measure of cybersickness. Graduate Theses and Dissertations, Iowa State University

Suma EA, Clark S, Krum D, Finkelstein S, Bolas M, Warte Z (2011) Leveraging change blindness for redirection in virtual environments. In: 2011 IEEE virtual reality conference. pp 159–166

Suma EA, Lipps Z, Finkelstein S, Krum DM, Bolas M (2012) Impossible spaces: maximizing natural walking in virtual environments with self-overlapping architecture. IEEE Trans Vis Comput Graph 18:555–564. https://doi.org/10.1109/TVCG.2012.47

Takada H, Fujitake K, Miyao M, Matsuura Y (2007) Indices to detect visually induced motion sickness using stabilometry. In: First international symposium on visually induced motion sickness, fatigue, and photosensitive epileptic seizures (VIMS2007). pp 178–183

Tanaka T, Kojima S, Takeda H, Ino S, Ifukube T (2001) The influence of moving auditory stimuli on standing balance in healthy young adults and the elderly. Ergonomics 44:1403–1412. https://doi.org/10.1080/00140130110110601

Templeman JN, Denbrook PS, Sibert LE (1999) Virtual locomotion: walking in place through virtual environments. Presence: Teleoperators Virtual Environ 8:598–617 . https://doi.org/https://doi.org/10.1162/105474699566512

Terenzi L, Zaal P (2020) Rotational and translational velocity and acceleration thresholds for the onset of cybersickness in virtual reality. In: AIAA scitech 2020 forum. American Institute of Aeronautics and Astronautics

Traschütz A, Zinke W, Wegener D (2012) Speed change detection in foveal and peripheral vision. Vision Res 72:1–13. https://doi.org/10.1016/j.visres.2012.08.019

Uliano KC, Kennedy RS, Lambert EY (1986) Asynchronous visual delays and the development of simulator sickness. Proc Hum Factors Soc Annu Meet 30:422–426. https://doi.org/10.1177/154193128603000502

Väljamäe A (2009) Auditorily-induced illusory self-motion: a review. Brain Res Rev 61:240–255. https://doi.org/10.1016/j.brainresrev.2009.07.001

Wang Y, Chardonnet J-R, Merienne F (2019a) VR sickness prediction for navigation in immersive virtual environments using deep long short term memory model. 1st IEEE VR workshop on immersive sickness prevention–IEEE virtual reality. Osaka, Japan, pp 1874–1881

Wang Y, Chardonnet J-R, Merienne F (2019b) Design of a semiautomatic travel technique in VR environments. IEEE virtual reality (VR). Osaka, Japan, pp 1223–1224

Whittinghill DM, Ziegler B, Case T, Moore B (2015) Nasum virtualis: a simple technique for reducing simulator sickness. In: Games developers conference (GDC)

Wibirama S, Hamamoto K (2014) Investigation of visually induced motion sickness in dynamic 3D contents based on subjective judgment, heart rate variability, and depth gaze behavior. In: 2014 36th annual international conference of the IEEE engineering in medicine and biology society. pp 4803–4806

Wienrich C, Weidner CK, Schatto C, Obremski D, Israel JH (2018) A virtual nose as a rest-frame– the impact on simulator sickness and game experience. In: 2018 10th international conference on virtual worlds and games for serious applications (VS-Games). pp 1–8

Williams B, Bailey S, Narasimham G, Li M, Bodenheimer B (2011) Evaluation of walking in place on a Wii balance board to explore a virtual environment. ACM Trans Appl Percept 8:19:1–19:14 . https://doi.org/https://doi.org/10.1145/2010325.2010329

Williams B, McCaleb M, Strachan C, Zheng Y (2013) Torso versus gaze direction to navigate a VE by walking in place. In: Proceedings of the ACM symposium on applied perception. Association for Computing Machinery, Dublin, Ireland, pp 67–70

Williams B, Narasimham G, McNamara TP, Carr TH, Rieser JJ, Bodenheimer B (2006) Updating orientation in large virtual environments using scaled translational gain. In: Proceedings of the 3rd symposium on applied perception in graphics and visualization. Association for Computing Machinery, Boston, Massachusetts, USA, pp 21–28

Wilson GF (2002) An analysis of mental workload in pilots during flight using multiple psychophysiological measures. Int J Aviat Psychol 12:3–18. https://doi.org/10.1207/S15327108IJAP1201_2

Wilson M (2016) The effect of varying latency in a head-mounted display on task performance and motion sickness. PhD Thesis, Clemson University

Xie X, Lin Q, Wu H, Narasimham G, McNamara TP, Rieser J, Bodenheimer B (2010) A system for exploring large virtual environments that combines scaled translational gain and interventions. In: Proceedings of the 7th symposium on applied perception in graphics and visualization. Association for Computing Machinery, Los Angeles, California, pp 65–72

Yang S, Schlieski T, Selmins B, Cooper S, Doherty R, Corriveau P, Sheedy J (2012) Stereoscopic viewing and reported perceived immersion and symptoms. Optom Vis Sci 89:1068–1080. https://doi.org/10.1097/OPX.0b013e31825da430

Yao R, Heath T, Davies A, Forsyth T, Mitchell N, Hoberman P (2014) Oculus VR best practices guide. Oculus VR 4:

Yokota Y, Aoki M, Mizuta K, Ito Y, Isu N (2005) Motion sickness susceptibility associated with visually induced postural instability and cardiac autonomic responses in healthy subjects. Acta Otolaryngol 125:280–285. https://doi.org/10.1080/00016480510003192

Young SD, Adelstein BD, Ellis SR (2006) Demand characteristics of a questionnaire used to assess motion sickness in a virtual environment. In: IEEE virtual reality conference (VR 2006). pp 97–102

Zhang R, Kuhl SA (2013) Flexible and general redirected walking for head-mounted displays. In: 2013 IEEE virtual reality (VR). pp 127–128

Zielinski DJ, McMahan RP, Brady RB (2011) Shadow walking: an unencumbered locomotion technique for systems with under-floor projection. In: 2011 IEEE virtual reality conference. pp 167–170

# Chapter 5
# Applications

**Abstract** The number of Virtual Reality (VR) applications in industry, gaming, in architecture, and cultural heritage, is increasing, yet they often are subject to cybersickness, unfortunately. The use of these techniques, which mostly emerged with the advent of 3D rendering techniques, concern driving or flight simulators for engineering design, manufacturing, and, since the 1980s gaming, using simulators or gaming now converge in hardware and software technologies as well as Virtual Reality Induced Sickness Effects (VRISE). A short overview allows to identify the commonly shared reasons of cybersickness, in navigation in the visuo-vestibular conflicts generated during controlled self-displacement. The now traditional Driver-in-the-Loop (DIL), as well as virtual mockup studies as well as Augmented Reality (AR) tools for Industry 4.0, are progressively completed with newer domains. Vehicle-in-the-Loop (VIL) simulation merges AR with real driving, and collaborative working employ increasingly realistic avatars interacting with each other. A last, new domain is the use of VR techniques to compensate foreseen motion sickness effects to be experienced in autonomous vehicles, which is another example of the advantage of being able to anticipate self-movement in virtual and real world, thanks to the perception of afferent information by the human brains.

## 5.1 Engineering Design and Manufacturing

Early industrial use of CAVEs, flight, and driver simulators, in some cases integrating Head-Mounted Display (HMD) systems dates back to the 1990s (see Chap. 1, Sect. 1.4.1). First use-cases were usually applied for Human–Machine Interface (HMI) design or validation in human factors departments, usually using driving or flight simulators, followed by mockup architecture or assembly studies. The latter do increasingly use immersive 3D installations (mostly CAVEs, more recently with Head-Mounted Display (HMD) helmets).

The use of driving or flight simulators has immediately brought out the undesirable simulation sickness effects during user experimentation. Even high-performance and motion-based simulators cause some sickness effects when the simulator movement

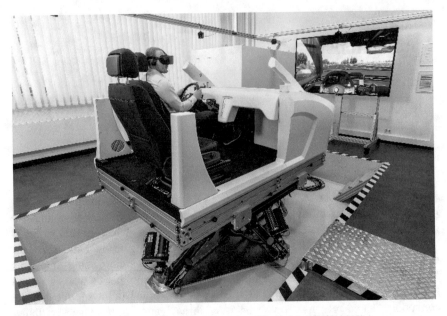

**Fig. 5.1** HMD-based driving simulator at Volkswagen (Hartfiel and Stark 2019)

exits the workspace designed to limit conflicts between visual and vestibular cues thanks to adapted Motion Cueing Algorithms (MCA). There is a large literature on MCA techniques (see Chap. 3, Sect. 3.2.2), and for a well-designed and strictly controlled set of user scenarios, often using onerous simulator setups, motion sickness may well be avoided.

For more limited, so-called static configurations, motion seats,[1] or G-belts[2] can be used to provide local kinesthetic cues for face value or, conversely, to induce generic motion solicitations, reducing the perception of specific motion cues, thus potential visuo-vestibular conflicts. For these limited systems, the immersion level must be coherent. A large Field Of View (FOV) display system with high-quality image rendering may reinforce the perception of conflicts with false motion cues, without providing external visual references which would allow the user to keep perceiving a stable external world.

CAVE installations are not suited to simulation of self-movement above a certain amount (typically, natural walking; see Chap. 3, Sect. 3.3) as they are not authorizing the use of motion systems. These systems are more apt for proximal perception, such as studying mockup design or ergonomics. CAVE-like simulators have been recently introduced that use stereoscopic 3D display systems all over the driver cab of a simulator (see Fig. 5.1). These simulators have the advantage of enhancing the

---

[1] D-BOX: https://www.d-box.com/en/professionals/expertise/race-simulation/.

[2] SimXperience, G-Belt Dual Axis Active Seat Belt Tensioning System: https://simxperience.com/en-us/products/accessories/g-beltactivebelttensioners/g-belt.aspx.

level of immersion and distance perception at the price of increased perceived visuo-vestibular incoherencies when the motion to be rendered is outside the workspace the system is able to render coherently.

Industry 4.0 features digital technologies and virtual and augmented reality technologies which are today largely deployed. Their use as tools to assist operators at the shop floor level is more and more widespread. Virtual reality tools, such as HMDs or CAVEs make it possible to design appropriate production lines to enhance productivity and efficiency. Furthermore, they help visualize and navigate through future factories at real scale, or simulate manufacturing processes such as assembly, thanks to multisensory feedback including haptics.[3] These possibilities should not obscure the fact that full immersion in a virtual environment can generate phenomena such as cybersickness. This happens when, for instance, navigation parameters are not well-tuned, or navigation techniques are not adapted to the context (see Chap. 4, Sects. 4.2 and 4.3). Augmented reality technologies are appropriate for on-site operations, such as guiding operators on manufacturing processes,[4,5] or maintenance operations[6]—sometimes assisted by a remote operator who can provide further information to the on-site operator. Compared to AR tablets, AR/MR helmets are more practical, as they allow operators to use both hands to perform their tasks in natural interactions. They can also be used in kitting operations,[7] or in on-site factory layout planning (Kokkas and Vosniakos 2019). However, an issue with helmets lies in the ergonomics of wearing such a device for extended periods, which can be tiring.

Many training applications are available today for Industry 4.0, concerning the use of new manufacturing systems, maintenance, safety procedures, and their learning. In situations involving robust safety procedures, VR allows training without endangering the trainees as well as their surrounding colleagues, which can represent a significant cost saving in terms of insurance. For instance, in logistics, forklift driving is a task that requires hours of training and VR can represent an interesting means to acquire the requested competencies. However, forklift training simulators may be similar to classical driving simulators with comparable effects to consider, such as sickness effects or issues related to speed and distance perception. If immersive (VR) HMDs are often used,[8] AR or MR helmets[9] are more adapted and are recommended. Indeed, they allow to overlay user instructions on top of the seen objects and environments while limiting cybersickness, since keeping vision of the outside visual

---

[3]ENSAM-Institut Image, Spidar: https://www.youtube.com/watch?v=qsoub_Bpfro.

[4]ZF Group, Smart factory with Microsoft HoloLens: https://www.youtube.com/watch?v=6pyiiO72ZwM.

[5]Immersion3D, Réalité mixte: Renault Trucks en route vers l'industrie 4.0 avec Immersion (Microsoft HoloLens): https://www.youtube.com/watch?v=RVafWc9Jqa8.

[6]Thyssenkrupp, Bringing new vision to elevator maintenance with Microsoft HoloLens: https://www.youtube.com/watch?v=biNebig1gUI.

[7]Inscape, Smart kitting at PSA with Inscape AR: https://www.youtube.com/watch?v=ndhnFCNwgpU.

[8]ENSAM-Institut Image, applications VR 1: https://www.youtube.com/watch?v=Lj3JYXExWUU.

[9]Fraunhofer FIT MARS, Remote Maintenance with Hololens: https://www.youtube.com/watch?v=1QFMPo5k6p0.

world with its stable visual references. In some cases, simple AR glasses are efficient enough, allowing for a natural use of the desired 3D information, thus preventing most cybersickness effects for all users.[10]

## 5.2 Simulation for ADAS and AD Development

To study and validate Advanced Driver Assistance Systems (ADAS), driving simulation, progressively equipped with CAVE-like or Head-Mounted Display (HMD) 3D systems, progressively becomes a well-known and largely used tool, as discussed earlier (Chap. 1, Sect. 1.4.1). In these systems, as the driver rarely undertakes large head movements, head tracking is still used seldom, which limits the impact of transport delay, the lag between driver actions and the rendered effects relative to the perceived environment modifications. However, lags between steering and vehicle motion represent a critical perturbation source, and conflicts between visual and vestibular sensorial information have made these systems the subject of intense cybersickness studies for many decades.

Several forecast studies recently emphasized the future impact of motion sickness for autonomous vehicles. Specifically, a significant number of autonomous vehicle users will experience motion sickness, since new compact, intermediate, or high-fidelity systems have been or will soon be put in use for ADAS and Autonomous Driving (AD) applications. Driver-in-the-Loop (DIL) simulation is then necessary to study driving delegation with frequent switching from autonomous to and back manual driving. Motion systems are used to prevent drivers from experiencing cybersickness (see Chap. 3, Sect. 3.2.2). Compact simulators use mostly limited vibration systems and more sophisticated installations include large 6 or 8 Degrees Of Freedom (DOF) motion systems (Fig. 5.2).[11,12] Chapter 4, Sects. 4.4, 4.5 and 4.6, provide more detailed information on cybersickness in driving simulation.

## 5.3 Vehicle-in-the-Loop Simulation

A seminal work, ahead of its time in the 1990s, published in 1992 (Sheridan 1992) and followed by an unpublished Vehicle-in-the-Loop (VIL) project at MIT, was carried out by Thomas B. Sheridan, a pioneer of robotics and remote control technology. He

---

[10]Vuzix Corporation, M3000 The Next Generation of Smart Glasses for Enterprise: https://www.youtube.com/watch?v=y6SGlOLVpg8.

[11]Groupe Renault, "ROADS", a new Renault driving simulator for autonomous vehicle, 2017: https://group.renault.com/en/news-on-air/news/roads-a-new-renault-driving-simulator-for-autonomous-vehicle/.

[12]BMW Group, BMW Group builds new Driving Simulation Centre in Munich, 2018: https://www.press.bmwgroup.com/global/article/detail/T0284380EN/bmw-group-builds-new-driving-simulation-centre-in-munich.

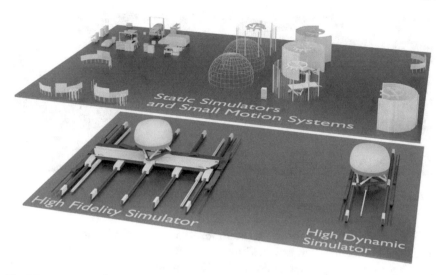

**Fig. 5.2** New BMW driving simulation center in Munich for development of autonomous driving systems, comprising 14 driving simulators

envisioned remote control of vehicles using VR technologies that were probably not sufficiently developed at the time to make its project viable. Nevertheless, the idea of using real vehicle driving to avoid the generation of false cues in motion rendering was used again by a couple of engineers at Audi (Bock et al. 2007). The authors claim that, while driving, if the synthetic outside traffic is visualized by the driver by means of an optical see-through HMD, motion sickness is avoided. Although no data were provided on motion sickness measures and results in sickness effects reduction, the setup allows for reproducible testing of driver assistance functions in critical traffic situations.

Other similar setups and experiments were proposed (Moussa et al. 2012), that involved the use of AR helmets; however, limitations to the usability of these techniques have not allowed their democratization. Unfortunately, reported simulation sickness (Karl et al. 2013), associated with longer reaction times, these early setups using HMDs, are insufficiently efficient tools for driving behavior studies.

As we have seen in Chap. 1 (Sects. 1.2 and 1.3.1), insufficiently short transport delays and consequent visuo-vestibular conflicts may still induce simulation sickness. Hence, later studies, using full (only virtual) VR helmets (Judalet et al. 2012) provides even more difficulties in producing sufficiently coherent visual and vestibular rendering of the real and virtual worlds. Recently, VIL systems were proposed with images directly projected on the windshield, a simple setup being using a projector and a screen placed ahead of the driver (Riedl and Färber 2015) (Fig. 5.3).

Future VIL systems may offer windshield AR visualization setups, making use of the already commercially available (Park et al. 2013) Head-Up Displays (HUD).

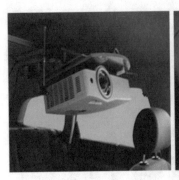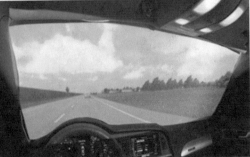

**Fig. 5.3**  On-board projector-based VIL setup (Riedl and Färber 2015)

The advent of massive simulation needs for autonomous vehicle and driving (AD) testing and validation, however, has brought new and enhanced VIL setups and will probably lead to significant deployment of Hardware-in-the-Loop (HIL) and VIL experiments (Horváth et al. 2019). Indeed, all the onboard driver and real traffic environments can be mixed with the thousands of necessary scenarios in different traffic situations for AD and AD-like ADAS testing and validation.

## 5.4  Architecture and Cultural Heritage Visualization

Architecture and cultural heritage are two close fields that have shown an interest in digital technology, particularly virtual reality and augmented reality. While the digital mockup has been adopted for several decades by the industry for engineering design, its concrete use in architecture and, more generally, the construction field is more recent. The specificity of the construction field is the high complexity of building processes, as they involve a large number of very different professions that traditionally execute highly manual tasks, which makes the management of building projects difficult. To facilitate exchanges and the management of building projects, Building Information Modeling (BIM) was imagined as a process to share a *digital representation of a built asset to facilitate design, construction, and operation processes to form a reliable basis for decisions* (ISO 19650–1:2018). Early concepts exist from the 1970s (Eastman et al. 1974), and first commercialized implementations were completed in the 1980s in Graphisoft's ArchiCAD architectural software (Forbes et al. 2010).

Several research projects have been initiated to push the use of virtual and augmented reality technologies in construction and cultural heritage. The objectives are to allow people to virtually visit full-scale buildings while virtually experiencing their physical properties, acoustic, and light rendering in real time to enable fast and reliable decision-making (Fig. 5.4).

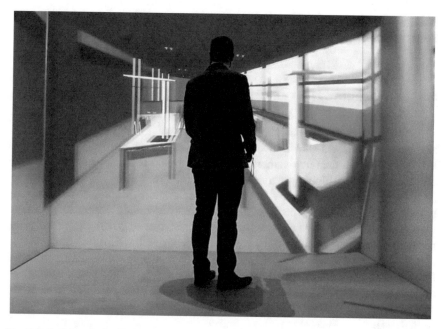

**Fig. 5.4** Building design review in a CAVE (Arts et Métiers)

VR and AR are seen as tools to help prototype, simulate construction, implement operation processes, detect potential issues, and allow customers to visualize the design better and define the best options before construction, which, by extension, also represents an impactful marketing tool (Whyte 2003; Raimbaud et al. 2019). As regards cultural heritage, these tools make it widely accessible in an entertaining yet pedagogical way; examples are Dassault Systèmes' Giza 3D application[13] and the 3D reconstruction of Cluny abbey by On-Situ[14]). Furthermore, VR and AR can facilitate heritage conservation and studies (Bekele et al. 2018) and make people conscious of the importance of preserving humanity's heritage (see, for instance, the 3D scanning implemented by Iconem of sites damaged or destroyed in Iraq and Syria[15]). Commonly required functionalities include navigation in large virtual mockups, interaction with virtual objects, collaborative working between people from different professions (see Sect. 5.6 below), and fast and reliable data management. With AR technologies such as interactive screens and smartphones, cybersickness does not occur since the user fully controls movements and while still seeing the surrounding real world, whereas it is much more likely to occur in immersive applications for real estate visits that can involve movements in constrained spaces with frequent turns or stairs ascending and descending (see Chap. 2, Sect. 2.3), in

---

[13]Dassault Systèmes, Giza 3D: https://www.3ds.com/stories/giza-3d/.

[14]On-situ, Maior Ecclesia: https://www.on-situ.com/fr/projets/60/maior-ecclesia/.

[15]Iconem, https://iconem.com/en/.

addition to interactivity issues linked to the navigation techniques used (see Chap. 4, Sects. 4.2 and 4.3).

## 5.5  Videogames

Videogames such as first-person shooter games involve fast navigation in immersive environments. As shown in Chap. 2 (Sect. 2.3.5), gamers usually experience less cybersickness than non-gamers since they develop strategies to move fast and accurately while developing spatial awareness abilities.

If the first-person perspective can be perceived as more thrilling, an alternative is to use the third-person perspective (which is usually an option suggested by default in games) to alleviate cybersickness effects (Monteiro et al. 2018). Specifically, the camera motion control in the third-person perspective allows for less frequent and abrupt movement when compared to the first-person perspective. Past work also found that in third-person viewpoint, players may look at a fixed point, such as the avatar's head, which causes less sickness (Clarke et al. 2016; Monteiro et al. 2018) since it has a similar effect as rest frames (see Chap. 2, Sect. 2.3.4, and Chap. 4, Sect. 4.3.4).

As discussed in Chap. 3 (Sect. 3.3), several hardware systems exist on the market to still benefit from the advantage of the first-person perspective while alleviating cybersickness effects by enabling real walking in a constrained space. However, these systems impose other constraints, such as being harnessed or using special shoes, which may impact user experience.

The convergence between gaming and industrial VR is not new, but the use of Unity or Unreal Engine from Epic games in industrial simulation software solutions has recently become overwhelming.[16,17] In this trend, one can foresee similar difficulties as those of industrial use when using immersive VR helmets. A variety of teleportation, blink,[18] or redirected walking techniques have been devised to avoid cybersickness (see Chap. 4, Sect. 4.2) and reduce the level of immersion (see Chap. 3, Sect. 3.3) when controlling self or avatar movements in the virtual environment. Nevertheless, although gamers are less sensitive to cybersickness, VRISE is still a major obstacle for a significant expansion of VR gaming and probably one of the

---

[16]Unreal Engine, CARLA democratizes autonomous vehicle R&D with free open-source simulator, 2019: https://www.unrealengine.com/en-US/spotlights/carla-democratizes-autonomous-vehicle-r-d-with-free-open-source-simulator.

[17]Bloomberg, Sony Invests $250 Million in Unreal Engine Maker Epic Games, 2020: https://www.bloomberg.com/news/articles/2020-07-09/sony-invests-250-million-in-fortnite-creator-epic-games.

[18]UploadVR, Cloudhead's "Blink" locomotion for VR is simple and robust, 2015: https://uploadvr.com/cloudhead-blink-vr-movement/.

reasons why the VR helmet market is still under the optimistic forecasts[19] made a couple of years ago.[20]

## 5.6 Collaborative Working and Avatars

In collaborative working, an important aspect is the representation of self and of the others (Schroeder 2012) (see also Chap. 4, Sect. 4.6). The sense of embodiment, defined as the sense of owning and controlling a virtual body (Kilteni et al. 2012), is a major research topic. A large body of literature exists on the influence of viewing avatars (Biocca 1997; Roth et al. 2016) that indicate its positive effects on presence (Kilteni et al. 2012). Specifically, avatar realism is of primary importance in collaborative working, as it can influence user experience (Bailenson et al. 2006). However, if differences between the users' own body and virtual body are too perceptible, users may experience the uncanny valley effect (Mori et al. 2012), which can affect presence. Avatar realism includes not only visual appearance but also behaviors (Steed and Schroeder 2015). Studies indicate that the absence of behavioral realism (e.g., the lack of face or gaze expressions) can impede social interactions (Roth et al. 2016) while not significantly affecting communication, which suggests that functional avatars may compensate for behavioral realism (Walther et al. 2015). An immediate advantage is that abstract avatars may suffice to foster social interactions within collaborative working, thus without needing high computer workload and intensive data transmission devices.

## References

Bailenson JN, Yee N, Merget D, Schroeder R (2006) The effect of behavioral realism and form realism of real-time avatar faces on verbal disclosure, nonverbal disclosure, emotion recognition, and copresence in dyadic interaction. Presence Teleoper Virtual Environ 15:359–372. https://doi.org/10.1162/pres.15.4.359

Bekele MK, Pierdicca R, Frontoni E, Malinverni ES, Gain J (2018) A survey of augmented, virtual, and mixed reality for cultural heritage

Biocca F (1997) The Cyborg's dilemma: progressive embodiment in virtual environments. J Comput Mediat Commun 3. https://doi.org/10.1111/j.1083-6101.1997.tb00070.x

Bock T, Maurer M, Farber G (2007) Vehicle in the loop (VIL)—a new simulator set-up for testing advanced driving assistance systems

Clarke D, McGregor G, Rubin B, Stanford J, Graham TCN (2016) Arcaid: addressing situation awareness and simulator sickness in a virtual reality Pac-Man game. In: Proceedings of the

---

[19]Road to VR, NVIDIA Claims 4 Million PC VR Headsets Sold, 2019: https://www.roadtovr.com/nvidia-claims-4-million-pc-vr-headsets-sold/.

[20]Business Insider France, THE VIRTUAL REALITY REPORT: Forecasts, market size, and the trends driving adoption, 2015: https://www.businessinsider.fr/us/virtual-reality-headset-sales-explode-2015-4.

2016 annual symposium on computer-human interaction in play companion extended abstracts. Association for Computing Machinery, Austin, Texas, USA, pp 39–45

Eastman C, Fisher D, Lafue G, Lividini J, Stoker D, Yessios C (1974) An outline of the building description system. Carnegie-Mellon University

Forbes LH, Ahmed SM, Ahmed SM (2010) Modern construction: lean project delivery and integrated practices. CRC Press

Hartfiel B, Stark R (2019) Influence of vestibular cues in head-mounted display-based driving simulators. In: Proceedings of the driving simulation conference 2019 Europe VR, pp 25–32

Horváth MT, Lu Q, Tettamanti T, Török Á, Szalay Z (2019) Vehicle-in-the-loop (VIL) and scenario-in-the-loop (SCIL) automotive simulation concepts from the perspectives of traffic simulation and traffic control. Trans Telecomm J 20:153–161

Judalet V, Glaser S, Kocher V, Charondiere D (2012) Virtual reality for real driving: a tool to fill the gap between simulators and test tracks. In: Proceedings of the Driving Simulation Conference

Karl I, Berg G, Ruger F, Farber B (2013) Driving behavior and simulator sickness while driving the vehicle in the loop: validation of longitudinal driving behavior. IEEE Intell Transp Syst Mag 5:42–57. https://doi.org/10.1109/MITS.2012.2217995

Kilteni K, Groten R, Slater M (2012) The sense of embodiment in virtual reality. Presence Teleoper Virtual Environ 21:373–387. https://doi.org/10.1162/PRES_a_00124

Kokkas A, Vosniakos G-C (2019) An augmented reality approach to factory layout design embedding operation simulation. Int J Interact Des Manuf 13:1061–1071. https://doi.org/10.1007/s12008-019-00567-6

Monteiro D, Liang H-N, Xu W, Brucker M, Nanjappan V, Yue Y (2018) Evaluating enjoyment, presence, and emulator sickness in VR games based on first- and third- person viewing perspectives. Comput Animat Virtual Worlds 29:e1830. https://doi.org/10.1002/cav.1830

Mori M, MacDorman KF, Kageki N (2012) The Uncanny valley [from the field]. IEEE Robot Automat Magaz 19:98–100. https://doi.org/10.1109/MRA.2012.2192811

Moussa G, Radwan E, Hussain K (2012) Augmented reality vehicle system: left-turn maneuver study. Transport Rese Part C: Emerg Technol 21:1–16. https://doi.org/10.1016/j.trc.2011.08.005

Park HS, Park MW, Won KH, Kim K-H, Jung SK (2013) In-vehicle AR-HUD system to provide driving-safety information. ETRI J 35:1038–1047. https://doi.org/10.4218/etrij.13.2013.0041

Raimbaud P, Lou R, Merienne F, Danglade F, Figueroa P, Hernández T (2019) BIM-based mixed reality application for supervision of construction. In: 1st IEEE VR workshop on smart work technologies—IEEE virtual reality. Osaka, Japan, pp 1903–1907

Riedl B, Färber B (2015) Evaluation of a new projection concept for the Vehicle in the Loop (VIL) driving simulator. In: Proceedings of DSC 2015 Europe driving simulation conference & exhibition, pp 225–226

Roth D, Lugrin J-L, Galakhov D, Hofmann A, Bente G, Latoschik ME, Fuhrmann A (2016) Avatar realism and social interaction quality in virtual reality. In: 2016 IEEE virtual reality (VR), pp 277–278

Schroeder R (2012) The social life of avatars: presence and interaction in shared virtual environments. Springer Science & Business Media

Sheridan TB (1992) Musings on telepresence and virtual presence. Presence Teleoper Virtual Environ 1:120–126. https://doi.org/10.1162/pres.1992.1.1.120

Steed A, Schroeder R (2015) Collaboration in immersive and non-immersive virtual environments. In: Lombard M, Biocca F, Freeman J, IJsselsteijn W, Schaevitz RJ (eds) Immersed in media: telepresence theory, measurement & technology. Springer International Publishing, Cham, pp 263–282

Walther JB, Van Der Heide B, Ramirez A, Burgoon JK, Peña J (2015) Interpersonal and hyperpersonal dimensions of computer-mediated communication. In: The handbook of the psychology of communication technology. Wiley, p 22

Whyte J (2003) Industrial applications of virtual reality in architecture and construction. J Inf Technol Construct (ITcon) 8:43–50

# Chapter 6
# Conclusion

**Abstract** Virtual (VR), Augmented (AR), or Mixed Reality (MR) form a continuum, also called XR. In this book, we attempted to define the underlying elements of these technologies and the relative experiences along with the generated sickness effects, called cybersickness or Virtual Reality Induced Sickness Effects (VRISE). The undesirable and, unfortunately, often experienced effects, previously studied in flight and driving simulators or, more recently, in virtual environments, are linked to various factors, such as conflicts between visual and kinesthetic (or vestibular) cues generated when moving in the virtual world. The main configurations of the usually proposed display and motion systems in VR inducing cybersickness were briefly recalled, to present their inherent VRISE generation features and the corresponding parameters, the user may tune for optimal use. A comparison was offered between virtual rooms (CAVE), Head-Mounted Display (HMD) helmets and simulators, and the various countermeasures—especially in VR, as AR technology is less subject to these effects—to help the readers use their installations efficiently. Following a short overview of user domains, which absorb an increasing part of our professional and social life, a brief analysis of the present trends was presented to provide an insight into the future evolution of Virtual Reality and cybersickness, and the way they may be experienced by the next generation of users.

## 6.1 Virtual Reality and Cybersickness

Virtual Reality (VR) and Augmented Reality (AR) techniques are significantly expanding today. Although VR already has had several setbacks, and even though a significatively lower market development was observed than forecasted, VR now seems to have become a mature technology. It is thus understandable that Virtual Reality Induced Sickness Effects (VRISE) or cybersickness is considered as a major issue. VR technology has various characteristics that are critical for sickness generation. One of them concerns the visual coherence between stereo vergence and eye accommodation. This issue is linked to today's rendering techniques and display technologies, as the 3D space is rendered by 2D images, provided for both eyes.

New techniques, using retinal display technologies may though change this situation in the future.[1]

The main configurations of the usually proposed display and motion systems in VR inducing cybersickness were recalled in this book briefly, to present the inherent VRISE generation characteristics and the corresponding parameters the user may tune with for optimal use. After a general presentation of self-motion perception and cybersickness, an overview of cybersickness reduction techniques was outlined, completed with best practices for VRISE avoidance.

Finally, for a synthetized set of application domains of engineering design, manufacturing, driving and vehicle-in-the-loop simulation, as well as architecture visualization and videogames, the main VRISE parameters were listed to help the readers optimize their installations, to prevent cybersickness. A brief comparison of VR, AR, CAVE, simulators, and collaborative environments helped to define the best-adapted configuration for the targeted applications.

## 6.2   How to Avoid Cybersickness

As cybersickness is a major issue in the usage of virtual reality technologies, dealing with proper strategies to prevent its effects is essential. Strategies are two-fold.

First, it is necessary to quantify cybersickness levels through either subjective (through questionnaires) or quantitative (through sensors and data logging) measurement means. A review of the existing methods with their pros and cons was proposed to enable choosing the appropriate methods. Choices must be made considering aspects such as the implementation costs, the time allocated to conduct the measurements or the relevance to the current problem.

Once cybersickness effects are measured, implementation of means to alleviate these effects should be devised. An extensive body of literature deals with the origin of effects, such as visual discomfort, stereoscopy issues, or visuo-vestibular conflict. A review of the several available solutions to improve immersive experience was then presented.

Specifically, light was shed on navigation as a typical use case where cybersickness is most likely to occur. Therefore, a strong part was devoted to different navigation techniques, including teleportation-based, motion-based, and controller-based techniques. Alternative solutions, consisting of adapting already well-known yet classical and simple techniques thanks to subtle modifications of what users see, were also presented.

As an example, adding visual references such as fixed objects within the users' field of view represents an efficient way to reduce visuo-vestibular conflicts without impacting much user immersion. The advantage of such adaptations are multiple: simple navigation techniques are features common to major development environments such as Unity or Unreal Engine, furthermore, adaptation techniques do not

---

[1] https://skarredghost.com/2020/07/30/mojo-vision-ar-contact-lenses/.

usually require strong programming efforts, and they can be deployed to many concrete situations involving navigation such as engineering and architectural design, and driving simulation.

Other means to reduce cybersickness effects were reviewed, including galvanic and auditory stimulation. Galvanic stimulation often comes up in the literature; however, no solution has been commercialized or deployed in concrete fields yet. Auditory stimulation is an attractive alternative due to the proximity with vestibular stimulation; hence it was largely used in past studies. The introduction of noise—either purely auditory or vibratory noise—can effectively impact the occurrence of cybersickness, and commercially available systems allow for their fast implementation to reduce cybersickness effects in situations such as driving simulation.

Best practices were finally detailed to provide a list of parameters to keep in mind when developing VR applications without VRISE effects, as these can originate from various factors. These practices are mainly suitable for VR since users are generally shielded from reality, which is not the case in AR where visual references are naturally present and cybersickness thus less likely to emerge.

## 6.3  Future Trends

Due to avatar's high level of presence and fidelity, new collaborative virtual environments will increasingly propose user avatars to provide a virtual world that is less and less distinguishable from real real-world users. As discussed earlier, links between the level of presence and cybersickness will be subject to further research. Recent developments also provide body vision with immersive Head-Mounted Displays (HMD), such as Oculus,[2,3] or video see-through wireless helmets such as Vive Cosmos[4] which reduce VRISE effects.

Sony have sold only 5 million of its Play Station VR until January 2020,[5] although more than 100 million PS4 was delivered as by March 2020,[6] which shows that there are still significant obstacles to the spread of VR helmets. Cybersickness is one of them, but the availability of sufficiently powerful computational units, integrated directly in HMD is another issue, because it limits image rendering quality without the use of cumbersome cables. There are already various wireless solutions in the market but with yet unsatisfactory streaming capacities. Sufficiently high-quality

---

[2]Oculus, Hand Tracking in Unreal Engine: https://developer.oculus.com/documentation/unreal/unreal-hand-tracking/.

[3]Nadav Grossinger, Israel Grossinger, Nitay Romano, Hand tracker for device with display, 2016: https://patents.google.com/patent/US9507411B2/en.

[4]CNET, HTC Vive Cosmos XR blends AR and VR using a snap-on faceplate, 2020: https://www.cnet.com/news/htc-vive-cosmos-xr-will-blend-ar-and-vr-with-a-snap-on-faceplate/.

[5]https://www.statista.com/statistics/987693/psvr-unit-sales/#statisticContainer.

[6]https://www.statista.com/statistics/651576/global-ps4-console-unit-sales/.

image rendering will be provided thanks to 5G streaming, changing our vision of not only virtual environments but also our everyday surroundings and, probably, our ways to live in them.

Some of the recent VR conferencing tools, such as Vive Sync,[7] already include Microsoft integrated collaborative VR working seances, with the possibility to pick up the most favored avatars, like gamers do, with selected appearance features, with or without VR helmets. Finally, even if virtual navigation remains linked to VRISE, the next generation of users may be less unaffected by the generated sensorial conflicts. Future users will move more and more easily in a virtual world at the price of being unable to capture sufficient sensorial information to evolve in human original nature, which meanwhile will progressively disappear due to all technological advances.[8] The authors give a rendezvous in a couple of years with the readers for more on these emerging technologies and corresponding research.

---

[7] Vive, VIVE Sync Feature Updates: June 2020, 2020: https://blog.vive.com/us/2020/06/23/vive-sync-feature-updates-june-2020/.

[8] Wikipedia, Ready Player One: https://en.wikipedia.org/wiki/Ready_Player_One.

# Index

**A**

Accommodation, vi, 9, 16, 20, 34, 47, 53, 71, 93, 120, 121, 143
Advanced Driver Aid Systems (ADAS), 18, 22, 136, 138
Aerospace, 14
Age, 31, 53, 94, 96
Auditory stimulation, 93, 114, 115, 145
*Augmented reality*, 3
Automotive, 13, 18
Autonomous vehicle, vi, 18, 22, 136, 138, 140
Autostereoscopy, 15, 63, 72, 73
Avatar, 7, 108, 121, 140, 141, 145

**B**

Binocular, vi, 20, 35, 68, 75, 120

**C**

Cave Automatic Virtual Environment (CAVE), v, 7, 11, 12, 14–19, 19, 107, 121, 134, 136, 139, 143, 144
Collaborative working, 7, 133, 139, 141
*Cybersickness*, 5
Cybersickness prediction, 102

**D**

Depth, vi, 9, 15, 16, 20, 21, 33, 73, 111, 117, 120
Display system, 10, 19, 20, 63–65, 68, 69, 71, 82, 134
Distance perception, 10, 16, 21, 32, 117, 120, 121, 135

Driver in the loop, 133
Driving simulators, v, 5, 14, 19, 20, 22, 23, 41, 48, 53, 78, 79, 85, 96, 112, 135, 137, 143

**E**

Embodiment, 7, 141
Engineering, vi, 15, 18, 120, 133, 138, 144, 145
*EXtended Reality (XR)*, 4

**F**

Field of view, vi, 6, 7, 9, 12, 21, 22, 43, 52, 54, 71, 76, 110–112, 117, 118, 121, 134, 144
Flight simulators, 77, 83, 95, 97, 133

**G**

Galvanic stimulation, 112, 113
Gaming, 7, 53, 54, 120, 121, 133, 140
Gender, 31, 48, 52
Gibson, 20, 23, 42, 121
5G streaming, 146

**H**

Head-mounted display, 1, 7, 9, 19, 68, 75, 87, 105, 110, 133, 136, 143, 145
Head movement, 20, 21, 38, 45, 46
Helicopter simulators, 17
Human factors, 22, 133

© The Editor(s) (if applicable) and The Author(s), under exclusive license
to Springer Nature Switzerland AG 2020
A. Kemeny et al., *Getting Rid of Cybersickness*,
https://doi.org/10.1007/978-3-030-59342-1

**K**
Kennedy, 5, 6, 18, 96


**L**
Light field, vi, 9, 63, 71, 73, 74, 76, 93, 120
Luminosity, 10, 67, 73


**M**
Manufacturing, 15, 73, 133, 135, 144
Measurements, 41, 99–101, 103, 111, 121, 144
*Mixed reality*, 4
Motion cueing, 22, 23, 63, 80, 81, 83, 114, 134
Motion parallax, 8, 11, 20–22, 47, 67, 71, 73, 117, 120
Motion rendering, 31, 39, 63, 77, 80–83, 137
Motion sickness, v, vi, 5, 7, 18, 31, 37, 43, 45, 48–54, 94–97, 100–102, 104, 112–114, 117, 118, 133, 134, 136, 137
Motion sickness susceptibility question-naire, 94


**N**
Navigation, v, vi, 6, 31, 48, 93, 94, 103–106, 109–112, 115, 117, 121, 122, 133, 135, 139, 140, 144, 146


**O**
Optic flow, 20, 31, 40, 110


**P**
Presence, 6


**R**
Reason, 5, 42, 48, 49, 52, 94
Rendering, 19, 20, 63, 93, 137
Retina, vi, 33, 34


**S**
Sensory conflict, 5, 49–52, 85, 114

Sheridan, 6, 136
Simulator sickness, 5, 6, 19, 48, 53, 96, 108, 112, 114, 119, 120
Simulator sickness questionnaire, 18, 94, 95, 111
Stereoscopy, vi, 6, 11, 16, 68, 70–72, 75, 120, 144
Sutherland, v, 8, 9, 19, 75


**T**
Teleportation, vi, 105, 106, 109, 121, 122, 140, 144
Training, 1, 18, 85, 135
Transport delay, v, 8, 9, 16, 19, 42–44, 46, 117, 136
Treadmill, 85, 86


**V**
Validity, 22, 50, 97, 104
Vection, 31, 41–43, 110, 114, 117
Vehicle in the loop, 136, 144
Vergence, 9, 16, 20, 33, 34, 47, 53, 71, 93, 120, 121, 143
Vestibular, vi, 5, 6, 20, 23, 31, 33, 36–44, 46, 48–51, 82, 83, 105, 106, 112–115, 117–119, 134, 136, 143, 145
Vestibulo-ocular reflex, 44–46
Videogames, 140
Virtual Boy, v, 1, 76, 119
*Virtual reality*, 3
Vision, 31
Visual cues, 20, 37, 82, 114
Visual references, v, 3, 7, 15, 16, 119, 134, 136, 144, 145
Visual rendering, 7–10, 15, 16, 22, 31, 63, 71, 73, 117–121, 133, 134, 138, 143, 145
Visuo-vestibular, 33, 40, 42, 63, 93, 115, 116, 121, 133–135, 137, 144
VR helmets, v, 5, 7, 9, 16, 65, 137, 140, 145, 146


**W**
Workbench, 14

Printed in the United States
by Baker & Taylor Publisher Services